# Current Topics in Microbiology
## and Immunology

**92**

Edited by

W. Henle, Philadelphia · P.H. Hofschneider, Martinsried
P. Koldovský, Düsseldorf · H. Koprowski, Philadelphia
O. Maaløe, Copenhagen · F. Melchers, Basle · R. Rott, Gießen
H.G. Schweiger, Ladenburg/Heidelberg · L. Syruček, Prague
P.K. Vogt, Los Angeles

# Natural Resistance
# to Tumors and Viruses

Edited by Otto Haller

With 22 Figures

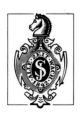

Springer-Verlag
Berlin Heidelberg New York 1981

Dr. Otto Haller
Institut für Immunologie und Virologie
der Universität Zürich, Gloriastraße 32 B
CH-8028 Zürich, Switzerland

ISBN 3-540-10732-0 Springer-Verlag Berlin Heidelberg New York
ISBN 0-387-10732-0 Springer-Verlag New York Heidelberg Berlin

# Table of Contents

*Indexed in Current Contents*

# Preface

Natural resistance is now coming to be recognized as a potentially important phenomenon in host defense against infection and malignancy. Genetically controlled resistance mechanisms are usually effective early in infection and before conventional immune responses are generated. Comparisons of experimental systems where natural resistance plays a prominent role demonstrate the complexities of the host defense mechanisms involved, as evidenced in the present volume. Nevertheless, some common components of genetic resistance are discernible and largely comprise natural killer cells, macrophages, and interferon. These and additional factors would seem to constitute a first line of defense in host resistance against both viruses and tumors. It is evident that considerable variation in the relative importance of distinct mechanisms may be found among various resistance systems and that, most likely, additional effector functions will be discovered.

Resistance to tumors and most viruses is under polygenic control, has a complex mode of inheritance, and depends on appropriately complex effector mechanisms. Instances, however, where a single gene locus determines resistance or susceptibility to a virus, as in the case of resistance to flaviviruses or influenza viruses, would seem to offer good prospects for elucidating the basic factors involved. Resistance to influenza virus would indeed seem to represent a comparatively simple situation: resistance is expressed at the host cell level, and interferon is its main mediator.

The present volume provides insight into current concepts of such resistance mechanisms. It contains contributions from distinguished laboratories presently engaged in relevant research in this field. A variety of experimental systems are analyzed covering genetic resistance in mice to flaviviruses, herpes simplex virus, lactate dehydrogenase elevating virus, influenza viruses and mouse hepatitis virus. Other chapters deal with interesting aspects of resistance to leukemogenesis and immunosuppression by Friend virus, with the biological significance of natural cell mediated immunity in viral infection and with tumor resistance and immune regulation by natural killer cells.

Zürich, April 1981                                    Otto Haller

# Genetically Controlled Resistance to Flavivirus and Lactate-Dehydrogenase-Elevating Virus-Induced Disease

MARGO A. BRINTON*

## 1 Introduction

The first demonstrations that a host gene could control resistance to disease induced by an animal virus were reported independently by *Lynch* and *Hughes* (1936) and *Webster* and *Clow* (1936). Subsequently this resistance was found to be specifically directed against flaviviruses. A number of other genes which confer resistance to other types of virus infections have since been identified (*Pincus* and *Snyder* 1975; *Bang* 1978). Different classes of viruses vary greatly in their mode and site of replication, and it would be expected that the mechanisms of action of various resistance gene products would also differ significantly. The strict virus specificity of host genetically controlled resistance indicates that the resistance gene products interact with unique molecular events characteristic of only one type of virus. Such a specific resistance mechanism acting at the cellular level constitutes a first-line host defense mechanism. However, the phenotypic expression of resistance genes on the whole-animal level can certainly be modified by the degree of functioning of other types of host defense mechanisms.

## 2 Genetically Controlled Resistance to Flaviviruses

More than 50 different flaviviruses have been identified to date by serologic means, and several of these are the cause of significant human morbidity and mortality worldwide. However, many of the molecular details of the flavivirus replication cycle are still poorly understood. Flaviviruses belong to the togavirus family, which also consists of alphaviruses, pestiviruses, rubivirus, and several unclassified viruses, including lactate-dehydrogenase-elevating virus (*Schlesinger* 1980). In general, togaviruses are characterized by a lipid envelope and an infectious single-stranded RNA genome. The various genera represented within the togavirus family are distinguished by differences in their modes of replication, by their fine morphological detail, and by their interaction with host resistance genes.

*The Wistar Institute of Anatomy and Biology, 36th Street at Spruce, Philadelphia, Pennsylvania 19104

*Webster* (1923), working with *Bacillus enteriditis* infection in a stock of randomly bred Swiss mice found that susceptibility varied greatly among individual mice. By selection and inbreeding, *Webster* (1933) developed bacteria-resistant (BR) and bacteria-suscepti-ble (BS) strains. Subsequent studies indicated that mouse strains resistant (VR) or sus-ceptible (VS) to Louping ill virus could also be selected, but that virus and bacterial resist-ance were inherited independently (*Webster* and *Fite* 1933, 1934). Mice resistant to Lou-ping ill virus were also resistant to St. Louis encephalitis virus (*Webster* 1937) and Russian spring-summer encephalitis virus (*Casals* and *Schneider* 1943). Since at the time of *Web-ster's* studies these viruses had not yet been classified (*Casals* and *Brown* 1954), the flavivi-rus-specific nature of the observed host-controlled resistance was not at first realized (*Sa-bin* 1953).

Genetically controlled resistance to yellow fever virus (YFV), another flavivirus, was independently observed by *Sawyer* and *Lloyd* (1931) among randomly bred Rockefeller Institute mice, by *Lynch* and *Hughes* (1936) among randomly bred mice of the "Det" strain, and by *Sabin* (1952a, b, 1954) in Princeton Rockefeller mice (PRI).

Within all known resistant mouse strains, "Det", BRVR, BSVR, and PRI, the flavivi-rus resistance is inherited as a simple autosomal dominant allele (*Lynch* and *Hughes* 1936; *Webster* 1937; *Sabin* 1952b). No other inbred mouse strains commonly used in laborato-ries have been found to possess the flavivirus resistance gene (*Darnell* et al. 1974). Using PRI mice as a source for the gene, another inbred resistant strain, C3H/RV, was created congenic to C3H/HE (*Groschel* and *Koprowski* 1965). C3H/RV and C3H/HE mice share common red blood cell antigens, and skin grafts are interchangeable between them. The development of the congenic C3H strains has allowed comparative studies of genetically controlled resistance to flaviviruses to be carried out against a low background of unrelat-ed variables. A study of wild mice caught in California and Maryland demonstrated the presence of the flavivirus resistance gene among wild mouse populations (*Darnell* et al. 1974) (Table 1). The finding that this resistance gene has continued to segregate within wild mice populations indicates that the gene may actually convey a selective advantage under natural conditions. However, which flaviviruses exert selective pressure on wild *Mus musculus* populations, other than possibly Powassan, is not yet known.

Factors such as the age of the host, its immune status, the degree of virulence of the infecting flavivirus, and the route of infection have been observed to influence the phe-notypic expression of the flavivirus resistance gene. However, no evidence has been re-ported which indicates that these factors are involved in the specific mechanism of resist-ance mediated by the product of the gene.

Resistant mice do support the replication of flaviviruses, but virus yields are lower and the spread of the infection is slower and usually self limiting as compared to suscept-ible mice (*Goodman* and *Koprowski* 1962a; *Darnell* et al. 1974). For instance, C3H/RV mice survive intracerebral injection of undiluted 17D-YFV, whereas 100% of C3H/HE mice die. The phenotypic expression of resistance can be overwhelmed by large doses of a virulent flavivirus given by the intracerebral route (*Goodman* and *Koprowski* 1962a). West Nile virus (WNV) can kill resistant mice after being injected intracerebrally, but 100–1000 times more virus is required to produce disease and death in resistant mice as compared to susceptible controls (*Vanio* et al. 1961; *Hanson* and *Koprowski* 1969; *Darnell* et al. 1974). The day of onset of disease symptoms is delayed in resistant mice, and the maximum virus titer in the brain is 2 to 3 logs lower than in comparable susceptible mice (see Fig. 1).

Table 1. Inheritance of resistance to yellow fever virus (YFV, strain 17D) in wild *Mus Musculus*

| Wild $(?)^a$ X C3H/He *(rr)* | |
|---|---|
| $F_1$ | |

| Wild parent | Surviving:dead[b] |
|---|---|
| $G3^{1\ c}$ | $0:9^c$ |
| $G3^2$ | 0:14 |
| $G3^3$ | 9:2 |
| $G4^1$ | 13:0 |
| $G4^2$ | 4:6 |
| $G5^1$ | 7:10 |
| $G5^2$ | 17:0 |

$F_1$ Survivors

↓

Resistant $F_1$ *(Rr)* X Resistant $F_1$ *(Rr)*[d]

↓

$F_2$

| | |
|---|---|
| | – |
| | – |
| | 7:3 |
| | 9:1 |
| | 7:2 |
| | 5:1 |
| | 6:0 |

| Total | 34:7 |
|---|---|

Reproduced with permission from *Darnell* et al. 1974
[a] Genotype
[b] Ratio of mice surviving challenge to those dying from it. Two litters of progeny from each parent were tested
[c] Two-month-old $F_1$ mice were given an intracerebral injection of 0.03 ml undiluted 17D-YFV
[d] Survivors were mated brother to sister approximately 2 months after their original infection

In susceptible animals the levels of neutralizing antibody and interferon which are produced in response to WNV infection are higher than in resistant ones; this corresponds to the higher titers of virus synthesized by susceptible animals (*Jacoby* et al. 1980; *Hanson* and *Koprowski* 1969; *Darnell* and *Koprowski* 1974). The in vivo expression of genetic resistance to flaviviruses requires an intact lymphoreticular system (*Goodman* and *Koprowski* 1962a; *Jacoby* and *Bhatt* 1976a, b; *Jacoby* et al. 1980). Immunosuppression of resistant animals with cyclophosphamide, sublethal X-ray irradiation, or thymus cell depletion converts a normally asymptomatic flavivirus infection into a lethal one. However, under such conditions the onset of sickness in resistant mice is delayed several days as compared to susceptible control mice, and the virus titers in moribund resistant brains are lower than in comparable susceptible brains. *Jacoby* and *Bhatt* (1976b) demonstrated that even though T-cell-depleted, flavivirus-infected resistant mice did produce detectable levels of hemagglutination-inhibiting antiviral antibody, they were not protected from lethal infections.

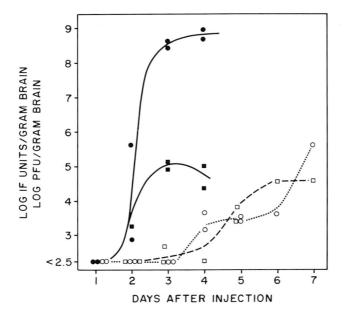

Fig. 1. Growth of West Nile virus (WNV) in the brains of susceptible C3H mice (●–●) and resistant C3H/RV mice (○–○). Interferon levels were also measured in brains of the C3H (■-■) and C3H/RV (□-□) mice. The intracerebral inoculum ($10^5$ PFU in 0.03 ml) was a WNV pool produced in $MK_2$ cells. (Reproduced with permission from *Hanson* and *Koprowski* 1969)

The clearance of WNV from the blood of resistant and susceptible mice has been found to be essentially complete by 10 to 12 h after an intraperitoneal injection of virus (*Goodman* and *Koprowski* 1962b). In susceptible mice, this clearance was immediately followed by a rise in the titer of infectious virus in the blood; virus levels in the blood remained high for at least 2 days. No such secondary viremia was detectable in blood from resistant mice (*Goodman* and *Koprowski* 1962b; *Groschel* and *Koprowski* 1965).

Cell cultures derived from various tissues of resistant mice produce lower yields of flaviviruses than do comparable cultures of cells from congenic susceptible mice. This phenomenon was first observed by (*Webster* and *Johnson* (1941), who studied the replication of St. Louis encephalitis virus in brain cell cultures from resistant and susceptible animals. *Goodman* and *Koprowski* (1962a) reported a similar difference in yield with WNV. Resistant brain cell cultures infected with WNV yielded 100-fold less infectious virus than did susceptible cultures. Cultures of spleen cells, peritoneal exudate cells, and embryofibroblasts from resistant animals displayed a similar diminished ability to support flavivirus replication when infected with either 17D-YFV or WNV (*Goodman* and *Koprowski* 1962a; *Vanio* 1963a, b; *Hanson* and *Koprowski* 1969; *Darnell* and *Koprowski* (1974). The differential ability to replicate flaviviruses was maintained in established cell lines developed from SV40-transformed resistant and susceptible embryofibroblasts (*Darnell* and *Koprowski* 1974). WNV adsorption and penetration occur normally in resistant cells, since the same percentage of cells show virus-positive immunofluorescence in resistant and susceptible cultures by 6 to 8 h after infection (*Darnell* and *Koprowski* 1974). Recent studies indicate that the level of flavivirus RNA and protein synthesis is significantly lower in resistant cells as compared to susceptible ones, indicating that inhibition of flavivirus replication within resistant cells occurs at an early step in virus replication (*Brinton* 1981b). We have isolated a number of temperature-sensitive mutants of WNV from persistently infected cultures of resistant and susceptible cells and are currently using these as tools for gaining a further understanding of the steps involved in flavivirus replication, as well as the differences in the virus-host interaction in resistant and susceptible cells.

The genesis of defective interfering (DI) virus particles, one type of viral deletion mutant, has been found to occur in cells infected with virtually any animal virus (*Huang* and *Baltimore* 1976) and seems to be controlled by host cell factors. Tissue culture experiments indicate that flavivirus DI particles are produced more readily and/or interfere with standard infectious virus replication more efficiently in resistant cells than in susceptible one (*Darnell* and *Koprowski* 1974). Assessment of the ability of serially passaged culture fluids from infected resistant and susceptible cell cultures to interfere with the replication of infectious homologous standard virus revealed that detectable interference was only observed with samples from resistant cells (Table 2). Since the ratio of defective to infectious particles determines the extent of interference, the lack of an observable interference by samples from susceptible cultures apparently was due to the presence of an insufficient number of DI particles to cause a detectable interference in the test. Susceptible cultures probably do produce DI particles as indicated by the cycling titer of infectious virus observed during serial undiluted passage in susceptible cells (Fig. 2). An identical decline in infectious vesicular stomatitis virus (VSV) was observed after serial undiluted passage in either flavivirus-resistant or -susceptible cell cultures, indicating that similar numbers of defective VSV particles are synthesized by both cultures and that the extent of interference is similar (*Huang*, personal communication).

The reduced yield of flaviviruses observed in resistant cultures and animals was not accompanied by an earlier or enhanced production of interferon (*Vanio* et al. 1961). As

Table 2. Interference between serial undiluted passage WNV and brain-produced WNV[a]

| Cell type | Moi of brain-produced WNV | 48 h WNV yield ($\log_{10}$ PFU/ml) | | |
|---|---|---|---|---|
| | | [b]Brain-produced WNV | [b]Brain-produced WNV plus 3rd passage T-MEF-HE WNV | [b]Brain-produced WNV plus 3rd passage T-MEF-RV WNV |
| T-MEF-RV | 1.82 | 2.7 | – | 1.9 |
| | 0.18 | 2.35 | 2.2 | 0.9 |
| | 0.018 | 1.0 | 1.75 | Undetectable |
| T-MEF-HE | 1.42 | 7.3 | – | 6.3 |
| | 0.14 | 6.6 | 6.5 | 5.75 |
| | 0.014 | 5.5 | 6.25 | 4.35 |

[a] WNV, West Nile virus. Reproduced with permission from *Darnell* and *Koprowski* 1974
[b] Titers of different virus preparations used for infection: brain-produced WNV = $10^{8.9}$ PFU/ml; 3rd passage T-MEF-HE WNV = $10^{4.5}$ PFU/ml; 3rd passage T-MEF-RV WNV = $10^{2.5}$ PFU/ml; T-MEF-RV = SV40 transformed resistant C3M/RV embryofibroblasts; T-MEF-HE = SV40 transformed susceptible C3M/HE embryofibroblasts

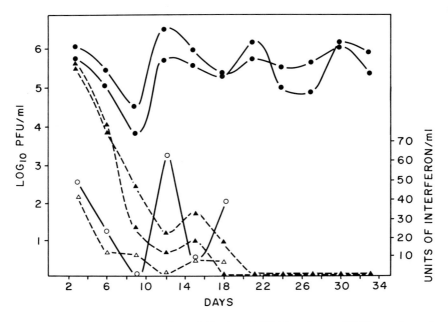

Fig. 2. Serial undiluted passage of West Nile virus (WNV) in cultures of SV40-transformed resistant and susceptible cells. Cultures were infected with WNV (10 PFU/cell) and culture media was transferred to fresh cultures every 3 days. Titers of WNV in transferred culture fluids from susceptible (●–●) and resistant (○–○) cultures and interferon from susceptible (▲–▲) and resistant (△–△) cultures are shown. (Reproduced with permission from *Darnell* and *Koprowski* 1974)

shown in Fig. 1, when 10- to 12-week-old C3H/HE (susceptible) or C3H/RV (resistant) mice were injected intracerebrally with $10^5$ plaque-forming units (PFU) of WNV, a dose sufficient to kill all the mice, the maximum levels of interferon measured in brain tissues were similar. Virus titers were characteristically lower in the resistant brains and rose later as compared to those in susceptible brains. Interferon production by WNV-infected resistant and susceptible cell cultures is low, but interferon levels were consistently higher in fluids obtained from susceptible cell cultures (*Darnell* and *Koprowski* 1974) (Fig. 2).

Vesicular stomatitis virus and Sindbis replicate equally well in flavivirus-resistant or -susceptible cells. The replication of these viruses was suppressed to an equal degree by treatment with crude interferon of both resistant and susceptible cultures, but interferon treatment caused an apparently greater suppression of WNV replication in resistant cultures than in susceptible ones (*Hanson* and *Koprowski* 1969; *Darnell* and *Koprowski* 1974) (Fig. 3). However, it must be remembered that the yield from non-interferon-treated resistant cells was already lower than that from susceptible cells. The apparent enhanced interferon mediated suppression of WNV production in resistant cells may be merely a synergism between interferon-induced inhibition and inhibition induced by the flavivirus resistance gene product.

In order to attempt to further clarify the role of interferon in the expression of flavivirus genetic resistance, the effect of pretreatment of animals and cell cultures with anti-interferon globulin was investigated. This study was done in collaboration with Drs.

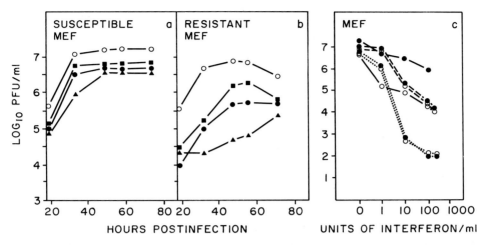

Fig. 3a–c. Inhibition of West Nile virus (WNV), Sindbis virus and vesicular stomatitis virus (VSV) production by crude interfeon in resistant and susceptible mouse embryofibroblasts (MEF). a Effect of interferon on WNV replication in susceptible cells. b Effect of interferon on WNV replication in resistant cells. Units of interferon used per ml of medium: (O–O) = 0 U/ml, (■–■) = 10 U/ml, (●–●) = 100 U/ml, and (△–△) = 1000 U/ml. c Comparison of interferon-mediated suppression of Sindbis, VSV, and WNV replication in susceptible (●–●) and resistant (▲–▲) cells. -, WNV; --, Sindbis virus, and --- VSV. (Reproduced with permission from *Darnell* and *Koprowski* 1974)

*Arnheiter, Haller*, and *Lindenmann*, employing sheep antimouse interferon (type I) antisera (AIF) obtained from Dr. *Gresser*. In the case of genetically determined resistance to orthomyxoviruses, injection of small amounts of AIF rendered resistant mice fully susceptible to lethal influenza virus infections (*Haller* et al. 1979). AIF-treated resistant animals showed a corresponding increase in virus production, so that virus titers similar to those in susceptible mice were observed. Normal sheep serum globulin (NSG) or AIF (neutralizing titer = $1.2 \times 10^{-6}$ against 8 units of mouse interferon) was diluted 1:3 with PBS, and 0.1 ml was injected into mice intravenously immediately before intracerebral injection of 17D-YFV ($10^3$ PFU/0.03 ml/animal). Two animals were killed at the indicated times after infection and their brains removed and frozen for subsequent titration (Table 3). Four animals from each group were observed throughout the course of the

Table 3. Virus titer in brain (PFU/brain)[a]

| Mouse strain | Treatment | Days after infection ($\log_{10}$) | | | |
|---|---|---|---|---|---|
| | | 3 | 6 | 9 | 12 |
| C3H/HE | NSG[b] | 2 [b] | 5 | 5 | – |
| | AIF | 2 | 5 | 6 | – |
| C3H/RV | NSG | – | 1 | 1 | 2 |
| | AIF | – | 1 | 1 | 2 |

[a] NSG, normal serum globulin; AIF, anti-mouse interferon serum. These were diluted 1:3 with PBS and 0.1 ml was injected intravenously immediately before virus was inoculated
[b] Titers represent average titer of virus in two brains homogenized and titrated separately

Table 4. Effect of AIF on mortality after YFV infection of C3H/HE and C3H/RV mice[a]

| Mouse strain | Treatment | Mortality | |
| --- | --- | --- | --- |
| | | Proportion | Mean day of death |
| C3H/HE | NSG[b] | 4/4 | 12 |
| | AIF[b] | 4/4 | 13.5 |
| C3H/RV | NSG | 0/4 | – |
| | AIF | 0/4 | – |

[a] Mice were given an intracerebral injection of 0.03 ml undiluted 17D-YFV (yellow fever virus) vaccine (titer = $10^4$ PFU/ml). NSG, normal serum globulin; AIF, anti-mouse interferon serum
[b] NSG and AIF were diluted 1:3 with PBS and 0.1 ml was injected intravenously immediately before virus was inoculated

infection (Table 4). In contrast to what was observed with myxovirus-resistant mice, AIF did not cause flavivirus-resistant C3H/RV mice to succumb to flavivirus infection (Table 4). Moreover, an increased production of flavivirus in the brains of resistant mice treated with AIF was also not observed (Table 3). AIF-treated resistant mice remained resistant when WNV was administered by the intraperitoneal route. In contrast, AIF treatment of susceptible C3H/HE mice led to a lethal infection after injection of a ten-fold sublethal intraperitoneal dose of WNV (Table 5).

Although it is not yet possible to describe the precise mechanism of action of the flavivirus resistance gene, some general statements can be made. Since a decreased yield of flaviviruses is observed for resistant cell cultures, the action of the gene is most likely at the cellular level. This assumption is further supported by the fact that lower titers of virus are also observed in resistant animals even after immunosuppression. Both interferon and DI particles interfere with virus replication at the intracellular level. Therefore, it would not be surprising to find that interferon and DI particle interference appear to be enhanced in resistant cells against flaviviruses simply because their effect is superimposed on viral replication processes already limited by the product of the resistance gene. Data indicate that the resistance gene product does not affect the attachment or penetration of flaviviruses but acts at an early replication step, resulting in a reduction in the level of virus-specific RNA synthesis.

Table 5. Effect of AIF on mortality after WNV infection of C3H/HE and C3H/RV mice [a]

| Mouse strain | Treatment | Proportion | Mean day of death |
| --- | --- | --- | --- |
| C3H/HE | NSG[b] | 0/3 | – |
| | AIF[b] | 3/4 | 14 |
| C3H/RV | NSG | 0/4 | – |
| | AIF | 0/4 | – |

[a] $10^7$ PFU/0.1 ml was given to each mouse by the intraperitoneal route. $LD_{50}$ for C3H/HE by the intraperitoneal route = $10^{7.5}$ PFU. WNV, West Nile virus; NSG, normal serum globulin; AIF, anti-mouse interferon serum
[b] NSG and AIF were diluted 1:3 with PBS and 0.1 ml was injected intravenously immediately before virus was inoculated

## 3 Genetically Controlled Resistance to Lactate-Dehydrogenase-Elevating Virus-Induced Paralysis

In 1970, *Murphy* et al. observed a fatal paralytic disease in C58 mice characterized by destruction of motor neurons in the brain stem and spinal cord. The virus causing this disease has recently been identified as a strain of mouse lactate-dehydrogenase-elevating virus (LDV) (*Martinez* et al. 1980). LDV normally produces a persistent infection in mice which is not characterized by any type of overt pathology. LDV is a small lipid-enveloped virus which contains a single-stranded infectious RNA genome and is considered to be in the togavirus family (*Brinton-Darnell* and *Plagemann* 1975; *Brinton,* 1981a). LDV infects only mice and replicates to high titers. LDV-infected animals maintain a lifelong viremia with virus present in the bloodstream within infectious immune complexes, but no clinical signs of an immune complex disease are manifested. A permanent increase in the plasma levels of certain enzymes, including lactate dehydrogenase (LDH) and isocitrate dehydrogenase, is also characteristic of LDV infection and is considered to result from an LDV-induced impairment of enzyme clearance by reticuloendothelial cells (*Riley* et al. 1960). The virus normally replicates in macrophages and macrophage-like cells in vivo and multiplies most efficiently in vitro in primary peritoneal exudate cultures (*Brinton-Darnell* et al. 1975). LDV infection induces subtle alterations in the functioning of the immune system such as a transient suppression of T-cell function during the first 2 weeks after infection (*Howard* et al. 1969; *Michaelides* and *Schlesinger* 1974) and an adjuvant effect on the production of antibodies to unrelated antigens (*Notkins* et al. 1966; *Mergenhagen* et al. 1967).

Several lines of evidence reported by *Martinez* et al. (1980) indicated that a strain of LDV is the etiologic agent of the C58 paralytic disease, which has been variously identified in the literature as age-dependent polioencephalitis (ADPE) (*Murphy* et al. 1970) and immune polioencephalitis (*Lawton* and *Murphy* 1973; *Sager* et al. 1973). Serum from animals with paralysis induces an increase in serum enzyme levels after injection into mice characteristic of an LDV infection (*Martinez* et al. 1980), and the infectivity titer of such sera as assayed by enzyme elevation endpoint or by paralysis induction endpoint was found to be identical. Physiochemical and morphological analysis also revealed the similarity of the C58 agent to LDV (*Martinez* et al. 1980). Further, even though previously isolated strains of LDV had not been known to cause an overt disease, they were found to possess a low level of paralytogenic activity for immunosuppressed C58 mice (Table 6).

The more paralytogenic LDV strain isolated from C58 mice may have been fortuitously selected by prolonged inadvertent passage in C58 mice as a contaminant of transplanted line Ib leukemia cell suspensions. Line Ib leukemia originated spontaneously in a 1-year-old C58 mouse in 1929 (*MacDowell* and *Richter* 1932) and has since been maintained by successive passages in C58 mice (*Murphy* et al. 1958). It is not known when the leukemic cell suspensions became contaminated with LDV (presumably from transfer of the leukemia cell suspension to a C58 mouse already persistently infected with LDV), but paralysis was not observed in C58 mice until the late 1960s (*Murphy* et al. 1970).

Although the LDV strains replicate in all inbred strains of mice tested and cause a nonsymptomatic persistent infection, LDV-induced paralysis has been observed in only two strains, AKR and C58 (*Duffey* et al. 1976b; *Martinez* et al. 1979). Further, AKR and C58 mice must first be immunosuppressed to become susceptible (*Duffey* et al. 1976b; *Murphy* et al. 1970). The genetic and immunologic factors involved in the induction of

Table 6. Test for paralytogenicity of LDV isolates in C58 mice

| Virus injected[a] | Incidence of paralysis in | | | |
|---|---|---|---|---|
| | 6-month-old mice | | 12-month-old mice | |
| | Proportion | Mean day ± SD | Proportion | Mean day ± SD |
| LDV-1 | 0/10 | | 9/11 | 16.9 ± 5.1 |
| LDV-2 | 1/10 | 18 | 6/10 | 15.2 ± 5.2 |
| LDV-3 | 0/10 | | 8/9 | 17.1 ± 5.2 |
| LDV-4 | 0/18 | | 6/19 | 19.0 ± 5.0 |
| C58 Agent | 10/10 | 12.1 ± 2.3 | 10/10 | 10.0 ± 0.5 |

[a] Mice were given cyclophosphamide 1 day before challenge with $10^7$ $ID_{50}$ of the indicated virus (as determined by enzyme elevation assay). LDV, lactate-dehydrogenase-elevating virus. Used with permission from *Martinez* et al. 1980

paralysis by LDV have been only partially characterized. The resistance of young adult C58 mice (up to 6 months) to induction of LDV-induced paralysis appears to be mediated by a thymus-dependent immune response which can be abrogated by neonatal thymectomy *(Duffey* et al. 1976a), immunosuppressive agents, or X-ray irradiation *(Duffey* et al. 1976b). Beginning at about 6 months, C58 mice spontaneously lose the function of a subpopulation of T cells and are then susceptible to LDV-induced paralysis without external immunosuppressive treatment *(Murphy* et al. 1970; *Murphy* 1979).

Virus infectivity titers in the plasma and tissues have been found to be maintained at higher levels after infection of immunosuppressed C58 mice with the C58 strain of LDV *(Nawrocki* and *Murphy* 1978; *Brinton* 1980a) (Fig. 4). Also, the injection of LDV immune complexes into immunosuppressed C58 mice does not lead to induction of paralysis, suggesting that antiviral antibody may be involved in the resistance to LDV-induced paralysis. Although an immunosuppressed state is required during the initial infection with LDV in C58 mice for the induction of paralysis to occur, an additional host genetic factor is involved; mouse strains which are completely resistant to paralysis induction apparent-

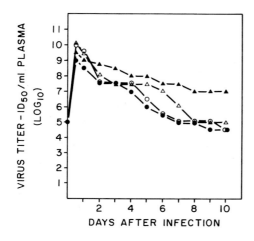

Fig. 4. Infectivity levels in plasma after infection of mice with the C58 strain of LDV. △–△, 3-month-old C58 mice; ▲–▲, 3-month-old C58 mice given 150 mg/kg cyclophosphamide 24 h prior to LDV inoculation; ○–○, 3-month-old Swiss mice; ●–●, 3-month-old Swiss mice given 150 mg/kg cyclophosphamide 24 h prior to LDV inoculation

Table 7. Susceptibility of inbred mice to paralytic disease

| $F_1$ hybrids | H-2 type | FV-1 type | Incidence of paralysis age (months) | | |
|---|---|---|---|---|---|
| | | | 6 | 9 | 12 |
| C58/wm X C3H/HeJ | k/k | n/n | 2/8 | 7/12 | |
| C58/wm X DBA/2J | k/d | n/n | 2/8 | 5/8 | |
| C58/wm X B10 | k/b | n/b | 0/26 | | 0/10 |
| C58/wm X B10.BR | k/k | n/b | 0/20 | | 0/14 |
| C58/wm X BALB/c | k/d | n/b | 0/11 | | 0/19 |

Used with permission from *Pease* and *Murphy* 1980

ly are not dependent on immunologic restriction of LDV, since the resistance of these mice is unaffected by immunosuppression (*Duffey* et al. 1976b; *Martinez* 1979). Preliminary analysis of the inheritance of host genes involved in controlling susceptibility to LDV-induced paralysis indicated that susceptibility might be controlled by two genes, one of which is linked to the H-$2^k$ loci (*Martinez* et al. 1979). However, recent breeding studies have revealed that susceptibility may not be linked to the H-$2^k$ loci. A correlation with the FV-$1^n$ allele has been suggested (*Pease* and *Murphy* 1980). From the $F_1$ data so far obtained, several genes appear to be involved in the inheritance of susceptibility to LDV-induced paralysis (Table 7). However, further breeding studies are necessary to delineate the number and type of host genes controlling susceptibility.

Electron microscopic examination of spinal cords from C58-LDV-infected immunosuppressed C58 mice revealed the presence of LDV-like virions within neurons. Previously, LDV was only known to replicate in macrophage-like cells. Virions were observed budding through neuron cytoplasmic membranes, but no cytopathic effect was obvious in virus-containing neurons. Virions have not yet been observed replicating in neurons within spinal cords of mice which are resistant to induction of paralysis after infection with the C58 strain of LDV. Virus infectivity was measured in spinal fluids at various times after infection. The C58 strain of LDV was readily detectable in the spinal fluid by 3 days after infection in both normal and immunosuppressed resistant and susceptible mice (*Brinton* 1980b) (Table 8). This LDV can apparently readily gain access to the central nervous system even during an infection which does not lead to

Table 8. Titer of C58-LDV in CSF[a]

| Mouse strain | Treatment | Days after infection | | |
|---|---|---|---|---|
| | | 3 | 6 | 9 |
| Swiss (r) | – – – | $6.5^b$ | 6.0 | 6.0 |
| Swiss (r) | Cyclo | 7.0 | 6.1 | 5.5 |
| C58   (s) | – – – | 7.65 | 7.0 | 7.0 |
| C58   (s) | Cyclo | 7.58 | 7.5 | 6.0 |

[a] LDV, lactate-dehydrogenase-elevating virus; CSF, cerebrospinal fluid
[b] $\text{Log}_{10}$ $\text{ID}_{50}$/ml

the induction of paralysis. Although these preliminary studies provide clues to the mechanism by which LDV can induce paralysis in a genetically susceptible immunosuppressed mouse, the exact sequence of events which produces lesions is not yet known. Further studies are necessary to determine the contribution to susceptibility of various T-cell subpopulations and the ability of neurons to replicate virus. It is not yet known whether neurons are damaged directly by virus replication or by attack by immune system components.

# 4 Summary

Resistance to flavivirus-induced disease is inherited in mice as a single autosomal dominant allele which shows no linkage to the H-2 loci. Resistant animals and cell cultures prepared from resistant animals produce two- to three-fold lower levels of flaviviruses than do comparable congenic susceptible mice or cell cultures. The product of the flavivirus resistance gene appears to act at the cellular level and, therefore, represents a virus-specific first-line defense mechanism. The resistance gene product does not affect the attachment or penetration of flaviviruses, but acts at an early step in virus replication, causing a reduction in the level of virus-specific RNA synthesis.

The genetic and immunologic factors involved in LDV-induced paralysis in mice have only partially been characterized. Although suppression of the function of a subpopulation of thymus-dependent cells does appear to be required prior to the induction of paralysis by LDV, an additional host genetically controlled factor is also necessary. Mouse strains which are resistant to LDV paralysis remain resistant after treatment with immunosuppressive agents. Further studies are needed to delineate the number and type of host genes which control susceptibility to LDV-induced paralysis. This system provides a unique opportunity to study the host factors involved in the production of a paralytic disease by a normally nonpathogenic virus.

# References

Bang FB (1978) Genetics of resistance of animals to viruses: I. Introduction and studies in mice. Adv Virus Res 23:269–348
Brinton MA (1980a) Lactate dehydrogenase virus (LDV) induced polioencephalitis of C58 mice. In: Boese A (ed) Search for the cause of multiple sclerosis and other chronic diseases of the central nervous system. Chemie, Weinheim, pp 222–229
Brinton MA (1980b) Genetically-controlled resistance to togaviruses. In: Skamene E, Kongshavn PAL, Landy M (eds) Gene control of natural resistance to infection and malignancy. Academic Press, New York, pp 297–303
Brinton MA (1981a) Lactate dehydrogenase-elevating virus. In: Foster HL, Small JD, Fox JG (eds) The mouse in biomedical research. Academic Press, New York
Brinton MA (1981b) Isolation of a replication efficient mutant of West Nile virus from a persistently infected genetically resistant mouse cell culture. J Virol (in press)
Brinton-Darnell M, Plagemann PGW (1975) Structure and chemical-physical characteristics of lactate dehydrogenase-elevating virus and its RNA. J Virol 16:420–433
Brinton-Darnell M, Collins JK, Plagemann PGW (1975) Lactate dehydrogenase-elevating virus replication, maturation, and viral RNA synthesis in primary mouse macrophage cultures. Virology 65:187–195
Casals J, Brown LV (1954) Hemagglutination with arthropod-borne viruses. J Exp Med 99:429–449
Casals J, Schneider H (1943) Natural resistance and susceptibility to RSSE in mice. Proc Soc Exp

Biol Med 54:201–202

Darnell MB, Koprowski H (1974) Genetically determined resistance to infection with group B arboviruses. II. Increased production of interfering particles in cell cultures from resistant mice. J Infect Dis 129:248–256

Darnell MB, Koprowski H, Lagerspetz H (1974) Genetically determined resistance to infection with group B arboviruses. I. Distribution of the resistance gene among various mouse populations and characteristics of gene expression in vivo. J Infect Dis 129:240–247

Duffey PS, Lukasewycz OA, Martinez D, Murphy WH (1976a) Pathogenic mechanisms in immune polioencephalomyelitis: quantitative evaluation of protective and pathogenetic effects of lymphoid cells. J Immunol 116:1332–1336

Duffey PS, Martinez D, Abrams GD, Murphy WH (1976b) Pathogenetic mechanisms in immune polioencephalomyelitis: induction of disease in immunosuppressed mice. J Immunol 116: 475–481

Goodman GT, Koprowski H (1962a) Study of the mechanism of innate resistance to virus infection. J Cell Comp Physiol 59:333–373

Goodman GT, Koprowski H (1962b) Macrophages as a cellular expression of inherited natural resistance. Proc Natl Acad Sci USA 48:160–165

Groschel D, Koprowski H (1965) Development of a virus-resistant inbred mouse strain for the study of innate resistance to arbo B viruses. Arch Gesamte Virusforsch 18:379–391

Haller O, Arnheiter H, Gresser I, Lindenmann J (1979) Genetically determined-interferon-dependent resistance to influenza virus in mice. J Exp Med 149:601–612

Hanson B, Koprowski H (1969) Interferon-mediated natural resistance of mice to arbo B virus infection. Microbios 1B:51–68

Howard RJ, Notkins AL, Mergenhagen SE (1969) Inhibition of cellular immune reactions in mice infected with lactic dehydrogenase virus. Nature 221:873–874

Huang AS, Baltimore D (1976) Defective interfering animal viruses. In: Fraenkel-Conrat M (ed) Comprehensive virology, vol 10. Plenum Press, New York, pp 73–116

Jacoby RO, Bhatt PN (1976a) Genetic resistance to lethal flavivirus encephalitis. I. Infection of normal and immunosuppressed congenic mice with Banzi virus. J Infect Dis 134:158–166

Jacoby RO, Bhatt PN (1976b) Genetic resistance to lethal flavivirus encephalitis. II. Effect of immunosuppression. J Infect Dis 134:166–173

Jacoby RO, Bhatt PN, Schwartz A (1980) Protection of mice from lethal flaviviral encephalitis by adoptive transfer of splenic cells from donors infected with live virus. J Infect Dis 141:617–624

Lawton JW, Murphy WH (1973) Histopathology of immune polioencephalomyelitis in C58 mice. Arch Neurol 28:367–370

Lynch CJ, Hughes TP (1936) The inheritance of susceptibility to yellow fever encephalitis in mice. Genetics 21:104–112

MacDowell EC, Richter MN (1932) Studies on mouse leukemia. V. A genetic analysis of susceptibility to inoculated leukemia of line I. Biol Zentralbl 52:266–279

Martinez D (1979) Histocompatibility linked genetic control of susceptibility to age-dependent polioencephalitis in mice. Infect Immun 23:45–48

Martinez D, Wolanski B, Tytell AA, Davlin RG (1979) Viral etiology of age-dependent polioencephalitis in C58 mice. Infect Immun 23:133–139

Martinez D, Brinton MA, Tachovsky TG, Phelps AH (1980) Identification of lactate dehydrogenase-elevating virus as the etiologic agent of the genetically restricted age-dependent polioencephalitis of mice. Infect Immun 27:979–987

Mergenhagen SE, Notkins AL, Dougherty SF (1967) Adjuvanticity of lactic dehydrogenase virus: influence of virus infection on the establishment of immunologic tolerance to a protein antigen in adult mice. J Immunol 99:576–581

Michaelides M, Schlesinger S (1974) Effect of acute or chronic infection with lactic dehydrogenase virus (LDV) on the susceptibility of mice to plasmacytoma MOPC-315. J Immunol 112: 1560–1564

Murphy WH (1979) Mouse model for motor neurone disease-immune polioencephalomyelitis. In: Behan PO, Rose FC (eds) Progress in neurological research. University Park Press, Baltimore, pp 175–193

Murphy WH, Wiens AL, Watson DW (1958) Impairment of innate resistance by triiodothyronine. Proc Soc Exp Biol Med 99:213–215

Murphy WH, Tam MR, Lanzi RL, Abell MR, Kauffman C (1970) Age dependence of immunologically induced central nervous system disease in C58 mice. Cancer Res 30:1612–1622

Nawrocki JF, Murphy WH (1978) Failure to eliminate antigen in an autoimmune central nervous system disease. Fed Proc 37:1120

Notkins AL, Mergenhagen SE, Rizzo AA, Scheele C, Waldmann TA (1966) Elevated γ-globulin and increased antibody production in mice infected with lactic dehydrogenase virus. J Exp Med 123:347–364

Pease JR, Murphy WH (1980) Co-infection by lactic dehydrogenase virus and C-type retrovirus elicits neurological disease. Nature 286:398–340

Pincus T, Snyder HW (1975) Genetic control of resistance to viral infection. In: Notkins A (ed) Viral immunology and immunopathology. Academic Press, New York, pp 167–187

Riley V, Lilly F, Huerto E, Bardell D (1960) Transmissible agent associated with 26 types of experimental mouse neoplasms. Science 132:545–547

Sabin AB (1952a) Nature of inherited resistance to viruses affecting the nervous system. Proc Natl Acad Sci USA 38:540–546

Sabin AB (1952b) Genetic, hormonal and age factors in natural resistance to certain viruses. Ann NY Acad Sci 54:936–944

Sabin AB (1953) Relationships between arthropod-borne viruses based on antigenic analysis, growth requirements, and selective biochemical inactivation. Ann NY Acad Sci 56:580–582

Sabin AB (1954) Genetic factors affecting susceptibility and resistance to virus diseases of the nervous system. Res Publ Assoc Res Nerv Ment Dis 33:57–67

Sager M, Lawton JWM, Murphy WM (1973) Serum transmissibility of immune polioencephalomyelitis in C58 mice. J Immunol 110:219–226

Sawyer WA, Lloyd W (1931) The use of mice in tests of immunity against yellow fever. J Exp Med 54:533–555

Schlesinger W (ed) (1980) The togaviruses. Academic Press, New York

Vanio T (1963a) Virus and hereditary resistance in vitro. I. Behavior of West Nile (E-101) virus in the cultures prepared from genetically resistant and susceptible strains of mice. Ann Med Exp Biol Fenn [Suppl 1] 41:1–24

Vanio T (1963b) Virus and hereditary resistance in vitro. II. Behavior of West Nile (E-101) virus in cultures prepared from challenged resistant, challenged backcross and non-challenged susceptible mice. Ann Med Exp Biol Fenn [Suppl 1] 41:25–35

Vanio R, Gavatkin R, Koprowski H (1961) Production of interferon by brains of genetically resistant and susceptible mice infected with West Nile virus. Virology 14:385–387

Webster LT (1923) Microbic virulence and host susceptibility in mouse typhoid infection. J Exp Med 37:231–244

Webster LT (1933) Inherited and acquired factors in resistance to infection. I. Development of resistant and susceptible lines of mice through selective breeding. J Exp Med 57:793–817

Webster LT (1937) Inheritance of resistance of mice to enteric bacterial and neurotropic virus infections. J Exp Med 65:261–286

Webster LT, Clow AD (1936) Experimental encephalitis (St. Louis type) in mice with high inborn resistance. J Exp Med 63:827–846

Webster LT, Fite GL (1933) Infection in mice following nasal instillation of Louping Ill virus. Proc Soc Exp Biol Med 30:656–657

Webster LT, Fite GL (1934) Distribution of virus of Louping Ill in blood and brain of intranasally infected mice. Proc Soc Exp Biol Med 31:695–696

Webster LT, Johnson MS (1941) Comparative virulence of St. Louis encephalitis virus cultured with brain tissue from innately susceptible and innately resistant mice. J Exp Med 74:489–494

# Resistance to Herpes Simplex Virus – Type 1 (HSV-1)

C. LOPEZ*

## 1 Introduction

In man herpes simplex virus-type 1 (HSV-1) has been shown to be the cause of several clinically important infections, including primary gingivostomatitis, herpes keratitis, and encephalitis (*Nahmias* and *Roizman* 1973; *Rawls* 1973). Clinically apparent as well as inapparent infections with HSV-1 have the capacity to become latent, i.e., the virus remains dormant in neurons but can become reactivated and cause an infection at a later date (*Stevens* 1975). Although the mechanism(s) involved in the establishment and maintenance of latency or in the subsequent reactivation of HSV-1 are not well understood, immunosuppression does not appear to be the trigger responsible for inducing the virus to reappear (*Spencer* and *Andersen* 1970; *Price* and *Schmitz* 1978). However, HSV-1 infections have been found to be especially problematic for those afflicted with congenital or acquired immunodeficiency disorders (*St. Geme* et al. 1965; *Aston* et al. 1972; *Lopez* and *Simmons* 1977). Thus, although the incidence of reactivated HSV-1 infections is not increased with immunosuppression, clearly the severity of reactivated infections is markedly exaggerated. These observations in man as well as a number of earlier animal studies (for example, *Nahmias* et al. 1969) have been taken as evidence that the immune response and especially the cell-mediated immune (CMI) system plays a primary role in resistance to these infections. Because of the complex nature of the pathogenesis of HSV-1 infections, resistance probably depends on several interacting subpopulations of cells (*Allison* 1974). The definition of these cells, their interactions, and their relative contributions will be important to future studies aimed at augmenting resistance to HSV-1. However, analysis in man of the various aspects of the immune response which might play an important role in the host's defense is complicated by the uncontrollable factors associated with the reactivation of latent herpes virus infections. Furthermore, man is genetically heterogenous and the capacity to delineate and dissect the genetically determined aspects of the host's defense system responsible for resistance to HSV-1 infections is limited.

*Sloan Kettering Institute for Cancer Research, 425 East 68th Street, New York, N.Y. 10021, USA

Because of the various shortcomings associated with the study of resistance to HSV-1 in man, much of our knowledge about host defense mechanisms has been generated by the study of animal (usually mouse) models. The mouse model of genetic resistance to HSV-1 described herein has certain advantages which make it especially useful for this study. Like other animal models, the investigator can control the various parameters of the experiments such as age and sex of the mice and route and concentration of virus inocula. In addition, the use of inbred strains of mice allows correlations of newly obtained data with that obtained from other, well-described genetic systems. Another advantage is that genetic tools can be applied to the study of resistance mechanisms. Thus, studies can be carried out to determine whether suspected resistance mechanisms segregate in crosses and backcrosses with genetic resistance. As will be shown below, the latter two advantages have been especially helpful in the study of the mechanisms involved in genetic resistance to HSV-1.

Although the study of animal models of resistance to HSV-1 offers certain advantages, the possible disadvantages must also be considered. One possibility is that an animal model may not resemble its human counterpart sufficiently to teach us much about the latter. For example, resistance to HSV-1 infections in mice could be mediated by mechanisms different than those found in man. This is especially true for the herpes viruses, since there appears to be evidence of coevolution of virus and its natural host. In effect, herpesviruses seem to have selected hosts capable of dealing with the virus infections. If inoculated into an animal of a related but different species, herpesviruses may cause violent, deadly infections. For instance, the B virus of rhesus monkeys is normally an innocuous virus found latent in kidney cells but which does not appear to cause disease in its natural host (*Hull* 1973). When accidently inoculated into man, this virus causes an almost uniformly fatal infection. The coevolution of virus and host seems to have selected for a natural host normally resistant to this virus. Study of resistance in the mouse might not reflect the resistance mechanisms which evolved in the rhesus monkey to the B virus or, for that matter, in man to HSV-1. One might, on the other hand, argue that the great susceptibility demonstrated in a different species might more clearly define the systems which evolved to determine resistance, i.e., susceptibility might not be partially compensaed for by another resistance mechanisms. The mouse model of resistance to HSV-1 has provided the rationale for developing new approaches to the study of resistance mechanisms in man. Fortunately, our studies of resistance to HSV-1 in man suggest that the mouse model has pointed us in an important and fruitful direction.

Resistance and susceptibility of the host are relative concepts which depend on such factors as age, sex, and condition of the host, size and route of inocula, virulence of the virus, and genetics of the host. In the experiments described in this chapter these factors were kept as constant as was reasonably possible. The age and condition of the mice was kept constant. In addition, most experiments have been carried out with mice inoculated intraperitonealy with highly virulent strains of HSV-1 (*Lopez* 1975; *Kirchner* et al. 1978a). In the studies of genetic segregation of resistance $10^6$ plaque-forming units (PFU) of virus were used as a challenge dose in order to clearly differentiate resistant from susceptible mice (*Lopez* 1980). Using these conditions we have been able to focus on the genetics of the host and evaluate resistance as an "all or none" phenomenon, even though this is clearly not the case.

## 2 Genetics of Resistance

Twelve inbred strains of mice have been tested for their capacity to resist infection with various doses of HSV-1 (strain 2931) (*Lopez* 1975). Adult (3–4 months old) male mice were inoculated by the intraperitoneal (i.p.) route with tenfold dilutions of virus. All mice were observed for at least 21 days, since earlier studies showed that mice which survived this period always survived for at least 3 months. Mice of the various strains appeared to be either resistant to $10^6$ PFU of HSV-1, moderately susceptible ($LD_{50}$ was about $10^3$–$10^4$ PFU), or very susceptible ($LD_{50}$ was about $10^1$–$10^2$ PFU). *Kirchner* et al. (1978a), using the WAL strain of HSV-1, confirmed these observations; they showed that inbred strains of mice could be categorized as resistant or susceptible. In both of these studies, mice of the C57BL background were found to be resistant while other strains were susceptible.

The earliest studies of genetic resistance were carried out using HSV-1 (strain 2931) which had been isolated from a patient with recurrent herpes labialis and had been passaged 30–40 times in Vero cell monolayers (*Lopez* 1975). In order to determine whether other strains of HSV-1 yielded similar results with the various inbred strains of mice, a number of new HSV-1 isolates and several well-studied laboratory strains were inoculated intraperitoneally into resistant C57BL/6 mice, moderately susceptible BALB/c mice, and very susceptible A/J mice. All of the virus strains tested demonstrated a similar pattern with these strains of mice: C57BL/6 mice resisted $10^6$ PFU of each of the virus strains tested, BALB/c were more susceptible, and A/J strain mice were susceptible to all but one strain of virus (*Lopez* 1975). HSV-1 (strain 2931) was found to be the most virulent of the strains tested and has been used throughout most of our studies. This strain of virus has been passaged routinely in vitro and has maintained its virulence. Kirchner's studies have been carried out with mouse-brain passaged HSV-1 (strain WAL) because tissue culture passage has yielded an avirulent strain of virus (*Kirchner* et al. 1978a). Although strain 2931 has not lost its virulence after tissue culture passage, HSV-1 (strain F) also appears to have lost virulence with passage in vitro (*Lopez*, unpublished work). These avirulent virus strains are not inert, since inoculation of mice with them induces resistance to subsequent challenge with virulent virus (*Lopez* 1975; *Kirchner* et al., to be published).

Studies by *Kirchner* et al. (1978b) also showed an interesting difference in susceptibility to HSV-1 of two very closely related strains of mice; C3HeB/FeJ and C3H/HeJ. The latter were found to be resistant to HSV-1 and to endotoxin, whereas the C3HeB/FeJ mice were susceptible to both. Since endotoxin was also found to induce lymphoid cells capable of replicating HSV-1 in susceptible but not resistant strains of mice, these data were taken to indicate an important role for endotoxin-stimulated cells in resistance to infection.

A series of studies were also carried out to determine the effect of route of inoculation on resistance to HSV-1 (*Lopez*, unpublished work). Tenfold dilutions of HSV-1 (strain 2931) were inoculated intraperitoneally, intravenously (i.v.), or intracranially (i.c.) into C57BL/6, BALC/c, and A/J mice (Table 1). When inoculated by the intracranial route, all strains of mice were susceptible to 10 PFU of virus suggesting that resistance to intraperitoneal or intravenous inoculation may be determined by the capacity of the host to interrupt virus spread to target tissue. The only difference found between intraperitoneal and intravenous inoculation was that A/J mice were much more resistant to the intravenous than to the intraperitoneal infection. Since A/J mice have been shown to

Table 1. $LD_{50}$ of HSV-1 (2931) inoculated by the intraperitoneal (i.p.), intravenous (i.v.), and intracranial (i.c.) routes

|          | i.p.                | i.v.            | i.c.           |
|----------|---------------------|-----------------|----------------|
| C57B1/6  | $> 10^6$ PFU[a]     | $> 10^6$ PFU    | $< 10^1$ PFU   |
| BALB/c   | $10^{2.34}$ PFU     | $10^{3.7}$ PFU  | $< 10^1$ PFU   |
| A/J      | $10^{1.0}$ PFU      | $10^{3.9}$ PFU  | $< 10^1$ PFU   |

[a] PFU, plaque-forming unit

have a defect of peritoneal macrophage function (*Boraschi* and *Meltzer* 1980), this might play a role in their increased susceptibility to intraperitoneal infection. Although all three strains of mice were found to be highly susceptible to an intracranial inoculation of HSV-1 (2931), our studies were not designed to determine whether there were differences between the strains of mice. Kirchner's studies, on the other hand, demonstrated small but significant differences between C57B1/6 and DBA/2 strains of mice when inoculated by the intracranial route (*Kirchner* et al. 1978b). The resistance patterns were similar to those obtained with intravenous inoculation and suggest that similar resistance mechanisms may be operative in the brain.

Our earlier studies (*Lopez* 1975), confirmed by *Kirchner* et al. (1978b), showed that $F_1$ crosses between resistant and susceptible mice were as resistant to HSV-1 infection as the resistant parent, indicating that resistance was a dominant genetic trait. Additional studies were carried out to determine the number of genes governing resistance. $F_1$ mice were backcrossed to the susceptible parents, which were either BALB/c or A/J mice, and the progeny were challenged with HSV-1. The results of these studies as well as the results of challenging an $F_2$ cross with HSV-1 indicated that two major genetic loci governed genetic resistance (*Lopez* 1980). Further backcrosses of resistant backcrossed mice to A/J mice indicated that other loci on the A/J background reduced resistance. Conversely, additional genes on the BALB/c background enhanced resistance (*Lopez* 1980). Therefore, although two major loci govern resistance, other minor loci influence this resistance.

Results from a number of studies have been taken to suggest that resistance to HSV-1 is immunologic in nature (*Nahmias* and *Roizman* 1973; *Lopez* 1978a). Since immune response genes governing the capacity to respond to certain antigens have been found to segregate with the major histocompatibility locus (the H-2) of the mouse (*Klein* 1975), studies were undertaken to determine whether the genes governing resistance to HSV-1 were likewise H-2 associated. A number of congenic mice were challenged with HSV-1: Mice with the resistant (C57B1) background and the H-2 of susceptible strains of mice were found to be resistant to HSV-1 (2931). Congenic mice on the susceptible (A/J) background into which had been introduced the H-2 of resistant mice were susceptible to the virus (Lopez, 1980). Thus, loci within the H-2 did not influence resistant or susceptibility. More recent studies (*Lopez*, unpublished work) suggest that resistance genes do not segregate with H-2 phenotype in backcross generations and, therefore, do not appear to be linked.

# 3 Thymus-Dependent Cells in Resistance to HSV-1

Herpesvirus infections are clearly much more severe in patients receiving immunosuppressive therapy (*Lopez* and *Simons* 1977; *Aston* et al. 1972; *Armstrong* et al. 1971). Similarly, resistance of mice to HSV-1 can be markedly diminished by treatment with immunosuppressive drugs (*Lopez* 1978a; *Nahmias* et al. 1969, *Zisman* et al. 1970, *Rager-Zisman* and *Allison* 1976, *Kirchner* et al. 1978a). These observations have been taken to suggest that the CMI system plays an important role in resistance to HSV-1 infections. The studies in man centered around patients receiving cytotoxic drugs for cancer (*Aston* et al. 1972; *Armstrong* et al. 1971) or for the prevention of graft rejection in renal, heart, and bone marrow transplant recipients (*Lopez* and *Simmons* 1977). Similarly, mice were immunosuppressed with cytotoxic drugs, antilymphocyte serum, or gamma irradiation in order to demonstrate increased susceptibility to HSV-1 infections. Since these treatments often suppressed the T-cell-dependent CMI response more profoundly than the humoral response, the CMI was thought to be required for resistance to HSV-1 infections. However, these various cytotoxic treatments are nonspecific and can impair the functions of a variety of T- and non-T cells. For example, *Schlabach* et al. (1979) recently showed that anti-thymocyte antiserum, in addition to its long-term suppressive activity against T cells, had a relatively short-term suppressive effect on host macrophage function which was specifically responsible for the increased susceptibility to HSV-1 in treated mice. Although earlier experiments with antilymphocyte serum and cyclophosphamide-treated mice demonstrated a breakdown of genetic resistance (*Lopez* 1978a), studies with athymic nude mice yielded very different results (*Lopez* 1978b, *Zawatzky* et al. 1979). Homozygous nude (*nu/nu*) mice have a congenital lack of a thymus and T-cells and, therefore, lack CMI responses such as the capacity to reject skin grafts or allogenic tumors (see *Klein* 1975). If the T-cell-dependent CMI response were required for resistance to HSV-1, then nude mice should be much more susceptible to HSV-1 than the normal controls. However, the nude mice were only slightly less resistant than controls in our study (*Lopez* 1978b) and slightly more resistant than controls in the study by *Zawatzky* et al. (1979). Clearly, the lack of a thymus and T cells did not significantly alter the resistance of these mice to HSV-1, indicating that these cells do not play an important role in genetic resistance.

# 4 The Macrophage in Resistance to HSV-1

The macrophage has also been thought to play an integral part in resistance to virus infections in general and to HSV-1 infection in particular. For example, *Mogensen* (1979) showed that genetic resistance to HSV-2-induced hepatitis in mice could be abrogated with silica and thus depended on macrophage function. (Although HSV-2 and HSV-1 are very similar viruses, the genetics of resistance to hepatitis is clearly different than genetics of resistance to HSV-1.) *Johnson* (1964) first showed that the age-dependent susceptibility of newborn mice to HSV-1 could be correlated with the inability of macrophages from the newborn mice to restrict replication of HSV-1 in vitro. Later studies showed that macrophage poisons impaired resistance to HSV-1 and that syngeneic adult macrophages conferred resistance to the normally susceptible neonatal mice (*Hirsch* et al. 1970). Because of these observations, attempts were made to diminish genetic resistance to HSV-1 by treating mice with macrophage poisons (*Lopez* 1978a) prior to infection with the virus. Silica and carrageenan were found to diminish resistance to HSV-1, although not to the level demonstrated by the genetically very susceptible mice.

The demonstration of an important role for macrophages in genetic resistance to HSV-1 prompted us to compare the capacity of macrophages from resistant versus susceptible mice to replicate virus in culture. These studies were patterned after those of *Stevens* and *Cook* (1971) which showed that macrophages from adult mice were able to restrict the replication of HSV-1 in vitro. Although the macrophages from the resistant strain of mice did not replicate HSV-1 as well as the macrophages from the more suscept-ible strains of mice, this capacity to sequester virus replication could not be correlated with resistance, since it did not segregate with resistance in $F_1$ crosses (*Lopez* and *Dudas* 1979). Macrophages from $F_1$ mice replicated HSV-1 as well as macrophages from the sus-ceptible mice, even though the $F_1$ mice were resistant to HSV-1. In fact, our study showed that the capacity of macrophages to replicate virus depended on the length of time in cul-ture and the inducing agent (if any) and much less on the genetics of the macrophage donor. These studies showed that the capacity of host macrophages to sequester repli-cation of HSV-1 (as evaluated in vitro) is not the mechanism of genetic resistance. However, this does not rule out another role for macrophages in genetic resistance.

## 5 Marrow-Dependent Cells in Resistance to HSV-1

When the properties of genetic resistance to HSV-1 were compared to those of genetic resistance to bone marrow allografts (*Cudkowicz* and *Bennett* 1971) a striking similarity was noted (*Lopez* 1978a). Specifically, (1) the distribution of inbred strains of mice within categories of resistant, moderately resistant, and susceptible were the same (*Cudkowicz* and *Bennett* 1971; *Lopez* 1975); (2) both resistance systems had been shown to be governed by two dominant, independently segregating loci (*Cudkowicz* 1975; *Lopez* 1980); (3) resistance in each case was diminished by cyclophosphamide, silica, or carrageenan (*Cudkowicz* and *Bennett* 1971; *Cudkowicz* and *Yung* 1977; *Lopez* 1978a); (4) both resistance systems matured rapidly at 3 weeks of age (*Cudkowicz* and *Bennett* 1971; *Lopez* 1978a); and (5) in each system resistance was conferred on susceptible mice by transplantation of bone marrow from resistant into susceptible mice (*Cudkowicz* and *Bennett* 1971; *Lopez* 1978a). There were only two differences noted: Resistance in each case was governed by two loci, both of which were required for resistance to HSV-1, while either of the two loci governing resistance to marrow allografts was sufficient for resist-ance to be demonstrated. In addition, gamma irradiation did not suppress marrow allo-graft resistance but greatly reduced resistance to HSV-1. However, since resistance to marrow allografts requires a 4-day assay and resistance to HSV-1 is evaluated over a 21-day period, the late effects of irradiation may be responsible for the decreased resistance to HSV-1. In other words, testing the resistance to marrow allografts 5 or 10 days after irradiation would probably demonstrate great sensitivity of marrow allograft resistance to gamma irradiation.

Because of the remarkable similarities between these genetic resistance systems, studies were undertaken to determine whether the marrow-dependent cell (M cell) which mediates resistance to marrow allografts also determined resistance to HSV-1. Studies by *Bennett* (1973) showed that treatment of genetically resistant mice with two doses of the bone-seeking radioisotope, strontium-89 ($^{89}$Sr), completely abrogated marrow allograft resistance. The $^{89}$Sr was taken up by bones and chronically irradiated the bone marrow with high-energy beta particles causing aplasia. In mice the spleen takes over the stem cell functions of the body and provides the cells required for humoral and cell-mediated immune responses (*Bennett* et al. 1976). Genetically resistant mice treated with $^{89}$Sr were found to be susceptible to the lowest concentration of HSV-1 tested ($10^3$ PFU), dying 5–7 days postinfection and thus at the same time as the genetically most susceptible strains of mice. Our study also showed that virus persisted in $^{89}$Sr-treated mouse spleen and liver tissue but not in the untreated mice. These observations indicate that the result of abrogation of M-cell function in HSV-1-infected mice is that the virus infection persists in the visceral tissues and travels to the spinal cord (*Lopez* et al. 1980). The latter is probably accomplished via the nervous system rather than hematogenously, since much less virus was found in brain than in spinal cord tissue (*Johnson* 1964).

Two other observations were made which were of interest. First, although the marrow-dependent cell shares certain similarities with macrophages, treatment of mice with $^{89}$Sr did *not* result in the HSV-1 causing a hepatitis. Since HSV-1 causes a hepatitis in mice whose macrophages have been impaired (for example, when treated with silica; *Mogensen* 1979), this particular macrophage function must have been relatively normal in order for no hepatitis to be induced. Second, infection of untreated, susceptible mice with HSV-1 causes a myelitis with infiltration of inflammatory cells into the spinal cord (*Walz* et al. 1977). In $^{89}$Sr-treated mice inoculated with HSV-1, virus could be isolated from the spinal cord and was detected by immunofluorescence, but an inflammatory response was not observed. Either mice were not studied late enough after infection or $^{89}$Sr treatment of mice impaired the inflammatory response normally induced by the virus infection.

Studies by *Haller* et al. (1977) and *Kiessling* et al. (1977) showed that natural killer cells (NK cells), first defined as a subpopulation of lymphoid effector cells which were capable of killing a variety of tumor target cells without prior exposure to the cells (see Chap.   in this volume), were also marrow dependent and their function could be abrogated by treatment with $^{89}$Sr. Because of these observations, an NK assay was developed to determine whether results with such an assay might correlate with resistance to HSV-1 in genetically resistant mice. Primary mouse embryo fibroblasts infected with HSV-1 were at first used as targets. Later, when we found that NK could be detected using UV-inactivated virus while at the same time reducing spontaneous release of radiolabel, our assay was routinely carried out with inactivated virus. Also, because of the high spontaneous release of $^{51}$Cr by mouse cells, the $^3$H-proline assay of *Bean* et al. (1976) was used. Our preliminary results suggest a strong correlation between this NK [NK (HSV-1)] and genetic resistance to HSV-1. Resistant strain mice, resistant F1 mice, and backcross mice which had earlier resisted challenge with $10^6$ PFU of HSV-1 (2931) all had spleen cells which responded significantly better than susceptible BALB/c and A/J mice (*Lopez* et al., to be published).

Studies by *Kirchner* and his collaborators (*Kirchner* et al. 1978c; *Zawatzky* et al. 1979) also strongly suggest that genetic resistance to HSV-1 depends on an "NK-like" cell which is capable of producing interferon when stimulated with HSV-1 antigen. These studies showed that 8 to 10 days after infection with live HSV-1 spleen cells from resistant mice made much more interferon when exposed to virus antigen than did the spleen cells of inoculated, susceptible mice (*Kirchner* et al. 1978c). Furthermore, when these investigators used a highly concentrated, band-purified antigen, similar results were obtained with resistant and susceptible mice which had *not* been infected with virus (*Zawatzky* et al. 1979). Thus, prior experience with HSV-1 was not necessary to show the difference between resistant and susceptible mice. Characterization of the subpopulation of cells which were responsible for making the interferon indicated that they were *non*-T cells, *non*-B cells, and *non*-macrophages (*Kirchner* et al. 1979) and thus might be NK cells.

## 6 Resistance to Human Herpesvirus Infections

As noted in the introduction, the mechanisms required for genetic resistance to HSV-1 infection in mice might not necessarily also play a role in resistance of humans to that virus infection. If, however, a similar mechanism can be found to play an important role in resistance of man, then the animal model would assume added significance. In fact, the results decribed above prompted us to develop an NK assay using HSV-1-infected human skin fibroblasts (*Ching* and *Lopez* 1979) to determine whether NK (HSV-1) could be correlated with resistance to herpesvirus infections in man. Although preliminary, our results suggest that the effector cells of NK (HSV-1) in man, like the M cell, are dependent on an intact bone marrow, since they were found to be very low in patients with marrow-deficiency conditions (*Lopez* et al. 1979; *Kirkpatrick* et al., unpublished work). In addition, study of patients with severe herpesvirus infections and patients susceptible to severe herpesvirus infections showed that these patients had NK (HSV-1) responses significantly lower than normal. Of special interest has been the observation that patients with Wiscott-Aldrich Syndrome (WAS) have very low (NK HSV-1) responses, since the immunologic deficiency associated with WAS also predisposes these patients to severe, life-threatening infections with HSV-1 (*St. Geme* et al. 1965). Study of the mouse model has thus directed us to the study of NK (HSV-1) in man and its relationship to resistance to herpesvirus infections. These studies suggest that similar mechanisms may be involved in resistance to HSV-1 in man as in the genetically resistant mouse. Further studies are required to document this relationship and to better understand this newly described effector system.

## References

Allison AC (1974) Interactions of antibodies, complement components, and various cell types in immunity against viruses and pyogenic bacteria. Transplant Rev 19:3–55

Armstrong D, Young LS, Meyer RD, Blevins AH (1971) Infectious complications of neoplastic disease. Med Clin North Am 55:729–745

Aston DL, Cohen A, Spindler MA (1972) Herpesvirus hominis infection in patients with myeloproliferative and lymphoproliferative disorder. Br Med J 4:462–465

Bean MA, Kodera Y, Shiku H (1976) Triitiated-proline microcytotoxicity assay for the study of cellular and humoral immune reactions directed against target cells grown in monolayer culture. In: Bloom BR, David J (eds) In vitro methods in cell-mediated and tumor immunity. Academic Press, New York, pp 471–480

Bennett M (1973) Prevention of marrow allograft rejection with radioactive strontium: evidence for marrow-dependent effector cells. J Immunol 110:510–516

Bennett M, Baker EE, Eastcott JW, Kumar V, Yonkosky D (1976) Selective elimination of marrow precursors with the bone-seeking isotope [89]Sr: implications for hemopoiesis, lymphopoiesis, viral leukemogenesis, and infection. J Reticuloendothel Soc 20:71–87

Boraschi D, Meltzer MS (1980) Defective tumoricidal capacity of macrophages from A/J mice. III. Genetic analysis of the macrophage defect. J Immunol 124:1050–1053

Ching C, Lopez C (1979) Natural killing of herpes simplex virus type 1-infected target cells: normal human responses and influence of antiviral antibody. Infect Immun 26:49–56

Cudkowicz G (1975) Genetic control of resistant to allogeneic and xenogeneic bone marrow grafts in mice. Transplant Proc 7:155–159

Cudkowicz G, Bennett M (1971) Peculiar immunobiology of bone marrow allografts. I. Graft rejection by irradiated responder mice. J Exp Med 134:83–102

Cudkowicz G, Yung YP (1977) Abrogation of resistance to foreign bone marrow grafts by carrageenans. I. Studies with the anti-macrophage agent seakem carrageenan. J Immunol 119:483–487

Haller O, Kiessling R, Orn A, Wigzell H (1977) Generation of natural killer cells: an autonomous function of the bone marrow. J Exp Med 145:1411–1416

Hirsch MS, Zisman B, Allison AC (1970) Macrophages and age-dependent resistance to herpes simplex virus in mice. J Immunol 104:1160–1165

Hull RN (1973) The simian herpesviruses. In: Kaplan AS (ed) The herpesviruses. Academic Press, New York, pp 389–426

Johnson RT (1964) The pathogenesis of herpesvirus encephalitis. II. A cellular basis for the development of resistance with age. J Exp Med 120:359–374

Kiessling R, Hochman PS, Haller O, Shearer GM, Wigzell H, Cudkowicz G (1977) Evidence for a similar or common mechanism for natural killer cell activity and resistance to hemopoietic grafts. Eur J Immunol 7:663–669

Kirchner H, Kochen M, Hirt M, Munk K (1978a) Immunological studies of HSV-infection of resistant and susceptible inbred strains of mice. Z Immunitaetsforsch Immunobiol 154:147–154

Kirchner H, Kochen M, Munk K, Hirt HM, Mergenhagen SE, Rosenstreich DL (1978b) Differences in susceptibility to herpes simplex virus infection of inbred strains of mice. IARC 24: 783–788

Kirchner H, Zawatzky R, Hirt HM (1978c) In vitro production of immune interferon by spleen cells of mice immunized with herpes simplex virus. Cell Immunol 40:204–210

Kirchner H, Zawatzky R, Engler H, Schroder CH (to be published) Studies of resistance of mice against herpes simplex virus (HSV). In: Skamene (ed) Genetic control of natural resistance to infection and malignancy (Abstr). p 17

Kirchner H, Peter HH, Hilfenhaus J (1979) Interactions between herpes simplex virus and the cells of the immune system. In: Proffitt (ed) Virus-lymphocyte interactions: implications for disease. Elsevier North Holland, New York, pp 259–265

Klein J (1975) Biology of the mouse histocompatibility-2 complex. Springer Berlin Heidelberg New York, pp 411–448

Lopez C (1975) Genetics of natural resistance to herpesvirus infections in mice. Nature 258:152–153

Lopez C (1978a) Immunological nature of genetic resistance of mice to herpes simplex virus type 1 infection. IARC 24:775–781

Lopez C (1978b) Genetic resistance to herpes simplex virus type 1 in the mouse is mediated by the M cell of allogeneic resistance. Fed Proc 37:1560

Lopez C (1980) Resistance to HSV-1 in the mouse is governed by two major, independently segregating, non-H-2 loci. Immunogenetics 11:87–92

Lopez C, Dudas G (1979) Replication of herpes simplex virus type 1 in macrophages from resistant and susceptible mice. Infect Immun 23:432–437

Lopez C, Simmons R (1977) Cytomegalovirus infections in renal and bone marrow transplantation. In: Touraine JP, Traeger J, Betuel H, Brochier J, Dubernard JM, Revillard JP, Triau R (eds) Transplantation and clinical immunology, vol IX. Proceedings of the Ninth International Course, Lyon. Excerpta Medica, Amsterdam Oxford, pp 17–24

Lopez C, Kirkpatrick D, Sorell M, O'Reilly RJ, Ching C (1979) Association between pre-transplant natural kill and graft-virus-host disease after stem cell transplantation. Lancet: 2:1103–1106

Lopez C, Ryshke R, Bennett M (1980) Marrow-dependent cells depleted by [89]Sr mediate genetic resistance to herpes simplex virus type 1 infections in mice. Infect Immun 28:1028–1032

Mogensen SC (1979) Role of macrophages in natural resistance to virus infections. Microbiol Rev 43:1–26

Nahmias AJ, Roizman B (1973) Infection with herpes simplex viruses 1 and 2. N Engl J Med 289: 667–674, 719–725, 781–789

Nahmias AJ, Hirsch MS, Kramer JH, Murphy FA (1969) Effect of antithymocyte serum on herpes-virus hominis (type 1) infection in adult mice. Proc Soc Exp Biol Med 132:696–698

Price RW, Schmitz J (1978) Reactivation of latent herpes simplex virus infection of the autonomic nervous system by postganglionic neurectomy. Infect Immun 19:523–532

Rager-Zisman B, Allison AC (1976) Mechanism of immunologic resistance to herpes simplex virus 1 (HSV-1) infection. J Immunol 116:35–40

Rawls WE (1973) Herpes Simplex Virus. In: Kaplan AS (ed) The Herpesviruses. Academic Press, New York, p 291–326

Schlaback AJ, Martinez D, Field AK, Tytell AA (1979) Resistance of C58 mice to primary systemic herpes simplex virus infection: macrophage dependence and T-cell independence. Infect Immun 26:615–620

Spencer ES, Andersen HK (1970) Clinically evident, non-terminal infections with herpesviruses and the wart virus in immunosuppressed renal allograft recipients. Br Med J 3:251–254

Stevens JG (1975) Latent herpes simplex virus and the nervous system. Curr Top Microbiol Immunol 70:31–50

Stevens JG, Cook ML (1971) Restriction of herpes simplex virus by macrophages. An analysis of the cell-virus interaction. J Exp Med 113:19–38

St Geme JW Jr, Prince JT, Burke BA, Good RA, Krivit W (1965) Impaired cellular resistance to herpes-simplex-virus in Wiscott-Aldrich syndrome. N Engl J Med 273:229–234

Walz MA, Price RW, Hayashi K, Katz BJ, Notkins AL (1977) Effect of immunization on acute and latent infections of vaginouterine tissue with herpes simplex virus types 1 and 2. J Infect Dis 135:744–752

Zisman B, Hirsch MS, Allison AC (1970) Selective effects of antimacrophage serum, silica and anti-lymphocyte serum on pathogenesis of herpes virus infection of young adult mice. J Immunol 104:1155–1159

Zawatzky R, Hilfenhaus J, Kirchner H (1979) Resistance of nude mice to herpes simplex virus and correlation with in vitro production of interferon. Cell Immunol 47:424–428

# Inborn Resistance of Mice to Orthomyxoviruses

Otto Haller*

## 1 Introduction

During evolution the vertebrate host has evolved a multitude of defense mechanisms to cope with virus infections. These are operative at several levels and range from simple physical barriers to complex structures such as the various parts of the immune system. Compared with acquired immunity, which has been so extensively studied, relatively little is known about resistance mechanisms in natural, genetically determined host defense against viruses.

Inborn resistance may be caused by barriers at several points in the virus-host interaction. Depending on the system studied, the following possibilities have been considered: Presence of humoral inhibitors in serum or secretions, lack of cell surface receptors,

---

*Institute for Immunology and Virology, University of Zürich, P.O.B., CH-8028 Zürich, Switzerland

abortive infection, release of noninfectious virus, production of defective interfering particles, induction of interferon, triggering of cellular, humoral, or secretory immune responses, pecularities of macrophages, and activation of natural killer cells.

In most cases, resistance to viral infections is under polygenic control and has a complex mode of inheritance. There are, however, instances where a single gene locus determines the degree of susceptibility to a virus. These simple situations should offer a practicable approach to elucidating some of the factors involved. In laboratory mice, single gene inheritance has been well documented in resistance to mouse hepatitis virus and to flaviviruses (reviewed by *Bang* 1978). Another good example is the resistance to the lethal effects of various orthomyxoviruses exhibited by mice carrying the dominant allele *Mx (Lindenmann* et al. 1963). Extensive studies exploring some of the factors mentioned above have been performed on the mechanisms by which the host gene *Mx* might confer resistance.

Here the main characteristics of inborn resistance to influenza virus will be reviewed and possible resistance mechanisms will be discussed in the light of earlier and more recent findings. The present data offer some new insight into the antiviral activity of interferon. They may therefore not only be pertinent to a variety of natural resistance systems operating via interferon mechanisms but may be equally relevant to a better understanding of interferon action in general.

## 2 The Experimental Model

A high degree of resistance to the lethal action of neurotropic influenza A virus was found by *Lindenmann* when mice of the inbred strain A2G were inoculated intracerebrally with an otherwise very regularly lethal doe of NWS virus (*Lindenmann* et al. 1963). The strain A2G originated at Glaxo Laboratories between 1942 and 1950 from an illegitimate mating between A and an unknown mouse. Inbreeding has been strict since 1950 for more than 100 generations (*Staats* 1976). Whereas A2G carries many alleles that differ from those in A/J, the major histocompatibility locus appears to be the same (H-$2^a$) (*Klein* 1975). In crosses between A2G and other strains, resistance is dominant, and backcrosses on many different genetic backgrounds yield 50% resistant animals, indicating the presence of a dominant allele (*Lindenmann* 1964, and unpublished observations).

From previous work, the inborn resistance to orthomyxoviruses found in mice carrying the dominant resistance allele *Mx* can be characterized as follows:

1. In homozygous animals resistance develops within 48 to 96 h of birth and in heterozygous animals, within 14 to 17 days (*Lindenmann* 1964). 2. Resistance is specific for members of the orthomyxo family. Mice bearing the resistance allele *Mx* are resistant to influenza viruses, but are as sensitive as control mice to several other viruses, such as flaviviruses, encephalomyocarditis (EMC) virus, or herpesviruses (*Lindenmann* et al. 1978; *Lindenmann* and *Klein* 1966). Although A2G mice have a certain degree of resistance to Sendai virus, it has not been established that this is due to the allele *Mx*, nor have other paramyxoviruses been extensively studied (*Lindenmann* and *Klein* 1966). 3. Resistance is expressed in various organs, namely in lung, in brain, and in liver against pneumotropic, neurotropic, and hepatotropic strains of influenza virus (*Lindenmann* et al. 1963; *Haller* et al. 1976). Virus replicates to 100 times higher levels in susceptible as compared to resistant mice (*Lindenmann* et al. 1963; *Haller* et al. 1976).

A liver-adapted variant of influenza A virus, TURH, has proved extremely useful for the analysis of inborn resistance of A2G mice. After intraperitoneal inoculation this hepatotropic virus, originally derived from an avian influenza A virus, grows rapidly in the livers of susceptible mice, causing acute liver failure and death within 2–3 days (*Haller* 1975). The livers of affected mice become pale yellow, swollen, and necrotic. The histologic examination of such livers reveals widespread and severe necrosis of hepatocytes. Resistant, *Mx*-bearing mice survive up to $10^4$ lethal doses (as measured in susceptible mice) of TURH. Histological sections of livers from infected resistant mice show only a few focal lesions with cellular infiltrates, which are self limiting. Hence, a plausible explanation postulated a particularly early or particularly efficient immune response.

# 3 Role of the Immune System for Resistance to Orthomyxoviruses

## 3.1 T-Cell-Deficient Nude Mice Express Resistance

If immune responses were responsible for resistance one would expect the expression of the resistance gene *Mx* to be impaired in mice immunologically not fully competent. Nude mice homozygous for the gene *nu* lack a functional T cell system (*Nomura* et al. 1977). We have therefore introduced the gene *Mx* into *nu/nu* mice, and we have investigated the phenotypic expression of resistance to various influenza A viruses in *Mx*-bearing nude mice (Table 1). Breedings were performed as previously described (*Haller* and *Lindenmann* 1974): Brother-sister matings among (*nu/nu* BALB/c × A2G)$F_1$ mice yielded an $F_2$ generation of which approximately 25% were phenotypically nude. Assuming independent segregation of the genes *Mx* and *nu*, 75% of these nude $F_2$ should carry the gene *Mx* either in homozygous or heterozygous form. If the nude phenotype did not prevent expression of virus resistance, 75% of these nude mice should resist an otherwise lethal challenge dose of virus. Table 1 illustrates that this was indeed the case with all virus strains tested. However, nude mice surviving virus challenge had significantly lower antibody titers than similarly infected nonnude controls. Furthermore, these animals, being immunologically not fully competent, were unable to clear the virus from the lungs and became chronic virus carriers as illustrated in Figure 1. Nude (Fig. 1a) and nonnude (Fig. 1b) littermates surviving 100 $LD_{50}$ of pneumotropic virus WS were compared as to anti-

Table 1. Resistance of nude F2 mice[a] to various influenza A viruses

| Group | Virus strain and route of inoculation[b] | Total No. of mice | Susceptible[c] No. | Resistant[d] No. | (%) |
|---|---|---|---|---|---|
| 1 | TURH   i.p. | 25 | 7 | 18 | (72%) |
| 2 | NWS   i.c. | 40 | 9 | 31 | (78%) |
| 3 | WS   i.n. | 125 | 32 | 93 | (74%) |
| 1–3 | Total | 190 | 48 | 142 | (74.7%) |

[a] 75% expected to be *Mx* carriers

[b] Hepatotropic avian influenza A virus TURH originally derived from A/Turkey/England/63 (Hav$_1$, Nav$_3$) was given intraperitoneally (i.p.). Human influenza A virus strains were the neurotropic variant NWS (H$_0$N$_1$) given intracerebrally (i.c.) and the pneumotropic variant WS (H$_0$,N$_1$) given intranasally (i.n.)

[c] Died of viral infection with signs of either neurologic disorder, pneumonia, or acute liver failure

[d] Survived virus challenge with 100 $LD_{50}$ for 4 weeks or longer

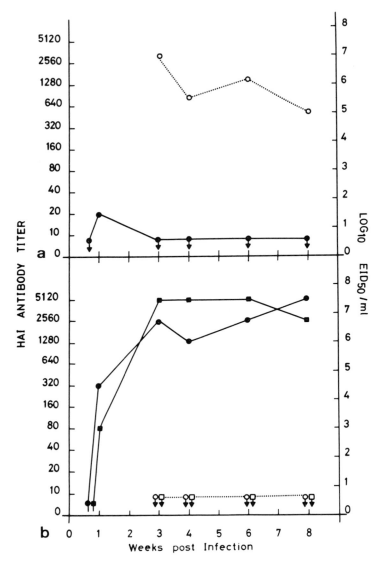

Fig. 1a, b. Antibody response and virus carriage in nude (a) and nonnude (b) mice (●, F₂ littermates, ■, A2G) after intranasal infection with 100 LD₅₀ of WS virus. Sera and lung extracts from five mice per group were assayed at the times indicated for hemagglutination-inhibiting (*HAI*) antibody titers (*closed symbols* and *straight lines*) and egg infectivity (*open symbols* and *broken lines*)

body response and virus carriage. In nonnude mice, hemagglutinating-inhibiting (HAI) antibody levels were significantly elevated after the 1st week of infection and reached high values during the 3rd week. Virus was never recovered from lung extracts beyond that time. In nude mice the situation was quite different: There was only a modest and transient rise in HAI antibody levels due to IgM production (*Haller* et al., unpublished work), and infectious virus could easily be detected in lung extracts for several weeks after infection (Fig. 1a).

We concluded that expression of resistance in mice carrying the allele *Mx* was independent of conventional T- and B-cell responses. Nevertheless, acquired immunity seemed to be indispensable to viral clearance and to recovery from disease.

## 3.2 B-Cell-Deficient CBA/N Mice Express Resistance

In T-cell-deficient *Mx*-bearing nude mice an early IgM response to the hemagglutinin of the challenge virus was regularly detected. The possibility existed that such T-cell-independent immune responses in the initial phase of viral infection were important for antiviral resistance. CBA/N mice carry an X-linked recessive B cell defect which prevents them from making antibodies to thymic-independent antigens (*Scher* et al. 1975a). Spleen cells from these animals have an impaired ability to participate in antibody-dependent cell-mediated cytotoxicity (*Scher* et al. 1975b). On the other hand, these mice display normal T-lymphocyte function as measured by T-cell cytotoxicity and skin graft rejection (*Scher* et al. 1975b) and exhibit high levels of natural killer cell activity (*Herberman* and *Holden* 1978). We have therefore investigated whether this particular immune unresponsiveness would modulate the expression of the resistance allele *Mx*. A2G mice were mated with CBA/N females homozygous for the X-linked recessive trait. The $F_1$ male progeny should express the B-cell defect whereas the $F_1$ female progeny should not; both sexes, however, would carry the dominant, autosomal gene *Mx* in heterozygous form. Table 2 shows that (A2G × CBA/N)$F_1$ male mice were resistant to lethal doses of our hepatotropic influenza virus strain. Clearly, the genetic trait of CBA/N mice was without influence on phenotype expression of the allele *Mx*.

## 3.3 Effect of Immunosuppression

Immunosuppression has been widely used to delineate the contribution of immune defense mechanisms to recovery from viral infections (*Allison* 1974; *Nathenson* and *Cole* 1970). Treatment of mice with cyclophosphamide has been shown to increase neurovirulence of influenza viruses in genetically susceptible animals (*Mayer* et al. 1973; *Miyoshi* et al. 1971). We have therefore tested the effects of cyclophosphamide and other

Table 2. Resistance of *Mx*-bearing mice with an X-linked B-cell defect to TURH virus

| Mouse strain | Sex[a] | B-cell defect | Mortality[b] |
|---|---|---|---|
| (A2GxCBA/N)$F_1$ | f | − | 0/8 |
| (A2GxCBA/N)$F_1$ | m | + | 0/8 |
| (A2GxCBA/J)$F_1$ | m | − | 0/8 |
| CBA/J | m | − | 8/8 |

[a] f = females; m = males
[b] Number of dead animals on day 7/total number of mice inoculated. Mice were infected i.p. with 100 $LD_{50}$ of hepatotropic influenza A virus, TURH

immunosuppressive drugs on the course of hepatotropic infection in resistant A2G mice. Resistance could not be abrogated by these treatments, although they prevented inflammatory infiltration by mononuclear cells at the site of viral replication and seemed to delay virus clearance (*Haller* et al. 1976). Similarly, *Fiske* and *Klein* (1975) have shown that immunosuppression by cyclophosphamide or X-ray irradiation did not influence the course of neurotropic infection despite the fact that these treatments rendered A2G mice unable to produce specific antiviral antibody or to generate cell-mediated delayed-type hypersensitivity responses.

# 4 Role of Macrophages in Antiviral Resistance

There is good evidence for a protective role of macrophages in viral infections. These cells monitor the main body compartments and are thought to represent a first line of antiviral defense. In the liver, Kupffer cells lining the sinusoids constitute an intact barrier protecting the adjacent parenchymal cells. Recruitment of mononuclear phagocytes is considered an important component of host defense. In both genetic resistance to mouse hepatitis virus (*Bang* and *Warwick* 1960; *Virelizier* and *Allison* 1976) and resistance to flaviviruses (*Goodman* and *Koprowski* 1961) macrophages from resistant but not from susceptible animals have been found to be capable of restricting virus replication in vitro. It has been proposed that the age-dependent development of resistance to herpes simplex virus in mice was due to functional maturation of the macrophage population after birth (*Johnson* 1964; *Hirsch* et al. 1970). We have therefore investigated the importance of macrophages for resistance to influenza viruses in our model system.

## 4.1 Macrophages Express Resistance Phenotype in Vitro

A strain of influenza A virus was adapted to grow in cultures of mouse peritoneal macrophages. This virus strain, called M-TUR, grew to high titers in macrophages from susceptible mice, thereby producing a marked cytopathic effect 36–48 h after infection (*Lindenmann* et al. 1978). It grew equally well in tissue macrophages such as Kupffer cells isolated from mouse liver (*Haller* et al. 1979b).

Whereas macrophages from genetically susceptible mice were fully permissive for influenza virus replication, freshly cultivated macrophages and Kupffer cells obtained from genetically resistant animals did not allow virus growth and showed no cytopathic effect (*Lindenmann* et al. 1978). Furthermore, a clear correlation between in vivo resistance of individual mice and in vitro resistance of their macrophages was found in segregation analyses using backcrosses between resistant (A/J × A2G)$F_1$ hybrids and susceptible A/J mice, indicating that resistance in vivo and macrophage resistance in vitro were two facets of the same phenomenon governed by the resistance allele *Mx*.

## 4.2 Macrophage Resistance and Resistance of the Intact Animal are not Causally Related

Since the correlation between in vivo resistance of individual mice and resistance of their macrophages in vitro was most striking, we speculated that macrophages, by interposing

Table 3. Resistance phenotype of chimeras repopulated with bone marrow stem cells from resistant (Mx/+) or susceptible (+/+) donors

| Type of chimeras | | Resistance phenotype[b] | |
|---|---|---|---|
| Donor | Recipient[a] | Macrophages | Intact animal |
| Mx/+ | +/+ | Resistant | Susceptible |
| +/+ | Mx/+ | Susceptible | Resistant |
| Mx/+ | Mx/+ | Resistant | Resistant |
| +/+ | +/+ | Susceptible | Susceptible |

[a] Irradiated with 850 rad and reconstituted with $3 \times 10^7$ viable bone marrow cells of sex-matched histocompatible donors

[b] Macrophage cultures were established from individual chimeras 12 weeks after marrow grafting and were tested for susceptibility to infection with macrophage-adapted influenza virus. Two weeks later the chimeras themselves were tested for resistance to influenza virus infection

themselves between the virus and its secondary targets, might be the main factor mediating resistance in vivo. To test this hypothesis, transfer experiments were performed in which macrophage precursors were adoptively transferred from resistant to lethally irradiated H-2 identical susceptible mice and vice versa (*Haller* et al. 1979b). These experiments are summarized in Table 3. Peritoneal macrophages taken 12 weeks after the transfer had the susceptibility pattern of the donor. The same was true for Kupffer cells in the liver, indicating that not only mobile macrophages but also tissue macrophages of the liver had been successfully replaced. Nevertheless, susceptibility or resistance of individual chimeric mice was according to the macrophage recipient and not according to the macrophage donor. Thus, animals of susceptible genotype died of infection in spite of harboring resistant macrophages, and animals of resistant genotype survived, although their macrophages were susceptible. We concluded that macrophage resistance and resistance of the animal did not seem to be causally related. The genetically determined capacity of macrophages to restrict influenza virus replication was obviously not a decisive factor in determining in vivo susceptibility or resistance.

As an aside, these experiments very nicely showed the bone marrow origin of the resident macrophage population in the liver. Previous work on macrophage origin in mouse radiation chimeras was based on differences in karyotypes (*Virolainen* 1968; *Howard* 1970) or differences in cell-surface markers (*Balner* 1963; *Godleski* and *Brain* 1972) between donor and host cells. To our knowledge, differences in genetically determined antiviral functions have not been previously used as markers in such studies. Since testing of *Mx* gene expression was not restricted to dividing cells (a serious limitation of chromosome marker techniques), our results on the bone marrow origin of Kupffer cells were most likely representative for the entire liver macrophage population. They corroborated previous findings in rodents (*Howard* 1970; *Godleski* and *Brain* 1972) as well as in man (*Gale* et al. 1978).

## 5 Natural Killer Cells in Host Defense Against Viruses

Viruses have been shown to induce high levels of natural killer (NK) cell activity in infected animals, possibly via induction of interferon (*Möller* 1979). After infection with lymphocytic choriomeningitis virus the increase in NK cell activity in mice correlated with interferon production. It preceded the appearance of virus-specific T killer cells (*Welsh* 1978). Although the significance of NK cells in acute viral infections is not yet clear, activation or recruitment of NK cells early in the infectious process and at the sites of initial virus replication might be a decisive factor controlling the degree of virus spread. A pertinent finding in this respect is the capacity of T-cell-deficient nude mice to reject otherwise tumorigenic cell lines when persistently infected with various RNA viruses, including measles, vesicular stomatitis virus (VSV), and influenza (*Minato* et al. 1979). There is evidence that NK-like cells are involved in natural resistance of certain inbred mouse strains against infection with herpes simplex virus type 1 (*Lopez* 1979).

Our own investigations have shown that inborn resistance to influenza viruses is expressed in nude mice known to exhibit high NK cell activity in spleen and blood and that resistance is highly dependent on interferon (see Sect. 6). Yet, we have failed to reveal a major role for NK cells in this form of resistance. Immunosuppressive treatments with cyclophosphamide, cortisone, whole-body irradiation and with silica, previously shown to greatly reduce NK cell activity in mice (*Kiessling* and *Haller* 1978), did not abrogate innate resistance of A2G mice (*Haller* et al. 1976; *Fiske* and *Klein* 1975). Furthermore, treatment with doses of radioactive strontium ($^{89}$Sr) that led to drastic impairment of NK cell function (*Haller* and *Wigzell* 1977), to abolishment of marrow allograft reactivity (*Bennett* 1973), and to abrogation of natural resistance against Friend virus leukemia (*Kumar* et al. 1974) did not affect A2G resistance.

In hemopoietic chimeras NK cell populations are known to be of donor genotype (*Haller* et al. 1977a). Enhanced resistance to herpes simplex virus type 1 (*Lopez* 1979) or to NK-sensitive tumor cells (*Haller* et al. 1977b) was transferable to suceptible animals by marrow stem cells from genetically resistant donors. However, attempts at transferring myxovirus resistance to genetically susceptible mice with marrow stem cells from resistant animals were not successful as already discussed. The chimera experiments of Table 3 would therefore argue against the possibility of NK cells being mediators of resistance to orthomyxoviruses.

## 6 Inborn Resistance to Orthomyxoviruses Depends on Interferon

Recent work with potent antiserum to type I mouse interferon has clearly demonstrated the beneficial role of interferon in the initial response of mice to different viral infections (*Fauconnier* 1970; *Gresser* et al. 1976a, b). That interferon would be involved in innate resistance of A2G mice to influenza virus seemed rather unlikely. Resistance was highly selective for orthomyxoviruses, whereas interferon is not thought to be virus specific. Furthermore, the amount of interferon produced after infection with influenza virus was constantly much lower in resistant mice as compared to susceptible controls (*Fiske* and *Klein* 1975; *Haller* et al. 1979a). However, when potent antiserum prepared against partially purified mouse interferon became available, it was found that treatment with this antiserum abolished resistance of A2G mice (*Haller* et al. 1979a).

Table 4 shows that treatment with sheep anti-mouse interferon globulin (AIFG) at the time of infection rendered genetically resistant mice fully susceptible to the lethal action of the hepatotropic influenza virus TURH. Virus titers in such mice reached levels similar to those observed in genetically susceptible animals. The same treatment also

Table 4. Effect of anti-mouse interferon serum on inborn resistance to hepatotropic influenza A virus[a]

| Mouse strain | Genotype | Virus titers[b] | | Mortality[c] | |
|---|---|---|---|---|---|
| | | NSG | AIFG | NSG | AIFG |
| A/J | (+/+) | 6.1 | 6.6 | 100% | 100% |
| A2G | (Mx/Mx) | 3.0 | 6.5 | 0% | 100% |
| (A/JxA2G)F$_1$ | (Mx/+) | 3.5 | 6.4 | 0% | 100% |

[a] Sheep anti-mouse interferon globulin (AIFG), neutralizing titer of $1.2 \times 10^6$, or normal sheep serum globulin (NSG) were given i.v. immediately before virus challenge. AIFG was prepared and supplied by Dr. *I. Gresser*, Institut de Recherches Scientifiques sur le Cancer, Villejuif, France
[b] $LOG_{10}$ EID$_{50}$/ml of heparinized blood pooled from five mice per group 48 h after infection
[c] Percentage deaths on day 7 after infection of four mice per group with 100 LD$_{50}$ of TURH virus i.p.

abrogated in vivo resistance to neurotropic and pneumotropic virus strains (*Haller* et al. 1979a).

Abrogation of resistance by AIFG lead to the expected changes in histopathology: Whereas only some local infiltrations by mononuclear cells were found in infected livers from A2G mice treated with normal sheep globulin, widespread hepatocellular necrosis was detected in AIFG-treated animals. These lesions resembled those usually observed in infected livers of genetically susceptible mice.

It has long been assumed that interferon plays an important role in host defense in viral infections (*Isaacs* and *Hitchcok* 1960). Interferon has been found to be a major component of the genetically determined resistance to mouse hepatitis virus in some strains of mice (*Virelizier* and *Gresser* 1978). The present findings indicate that interferon is an integral and important part of the inborn resistance to influenza virus in mice carrying the gene *Mx*.

## 7 Interferon-Dependent Resistance Develops in Fetal Mouse Brain Cells During Differentiation in Aggregating Cultures

Attempts to demonstrate resistance in monolayer cultures of brain or kidney cells have never been successful (*Rusanova* and *Soloview* 1966; *Vallbracht* 1977; and unpublished works). These cells are usually obtained from embryonal or neonatal animals which themselves do not yet exhibit the full resistance of the adult. Macrophages from adult animals differ from fetal cells in that they preserve a high degree of cellular differentiation in culture. We therefore speculated that some maturation step was needed for phenotype expression of the resistance gene *Mx*. If this were the case, it should be possible to analyze the development of antiviral resistance in a culture system allowing cell maturation in vitro.

Aggregating cultures of mechanically dissociated fetal brain cells represent such a differentiation model (*Honegger* and *Richelson* 1976; *Honegger* et al. 1979). Cells in aggregating cultures undergo morphological and biochemical changes that mimic normal brain development in vivo. Within 25 to 30 days of culturing, they mature from a completely undifferentiated state to a population of morphologically mature neurons, astrocytes, and oligodendrocytes (*Trapp* et al. 1979). Correspondingly, specific activity of various neuron-specific enzymes increases from low levels during the 1st week to maximal levels resembling those usually found in adult tissue in vivo after the 3rd week of culture (*Honegger* and *Richelson* 1976; *Honegger* et al. 1979).

To test our hypothesis, we investigated whether aggregating cultures of A2G brain cells would express the resistance phenotype as a consequence of age-dependent maturation in vitro (*Haller* and *Honegger*, to be published). Excised brains from 16-day-old mouse fetuses of susceptible or resistant genotype were mechanically dissociated into single cells, incubated in nutrient medium, and grown in rotation-mediated aggregate culture as described by *Honegger* and *Richelson* (1976). Aggregates were allowed to differentiate for 6 to 40 days in vitro before infection with NWS, the Stuart-Harris strain of neurotropic influenza A virus (*Stuart-Harris* 1939) originally used in the discovery of inborn resistance of A2G mice (*Lindenmann* 1962). NWS virus grew to high titers in cultures of susceptible A/J cells of all ages tested. In contrast, NWS multiplication was restricted in differentiated A2G aggregates kept for 32 days in culture. Figure 2 shows the growth curves of NWS in 32-day-old susceptible and resistant aggregates. Both A2G and A/J aggregating brain cells supported viral growth, but maximum titers in A2G aggregates were about 1000 times lower than those in A/J aggregates. This characteristic log 2 to log 3 difference in maximal virus yields between susceptible and resistant cultures was detectable with high and low multiplicities of infection and was in complete agreement with previous in vivo data on viral growth in brains of normal (*Lindenmann* et al. 1963) or immunosuppressed A2G mice (*Fiske* and *Klein* 1975).

The histopathology of infected brain cell aggregates confirmed the present observations: NWS infection of A/J brain cell aggregates led to a pronounced cytopathic effect within 72 h characterized by widespread cellular degeneration with pyknosis and karyorrhexis. Immunofluorescent staining of frozen sections revealed the presence of large amounts of virus-specific antigens scattered thoughout the aggregates. In contrast, necrosis in infected 32-day aggregates of A2G brain cells was confined to minute foci lo-

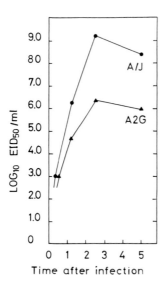

Fig. 2. Growth of NWS virus in brain cell aggregates established from genetically susceptible A/J mice (●—●) or from resistant A2G mice homozygous for the allele *Mx* (▲—▲). 32 day aggregates from two culture flasks were pooled, homogenized, and assayed for infectivity in 10-day-old embryonated chicken eggs at the times indicated. $EID_{50}$, mean egg infective dose

calized mainly at the periphery of the aggregates where specific fluorescence of single cells was detectable. These observations are in good agreement with immunofluorescent findings in brain sections of A2G mice infected intracerebrally with neuropathogenic influenza A virus (*Fiske* and *Klein* 1975).

Since adult but not newborn A2G mice survived infection with neurotropic influenza virus strains (capable of causing fatal encephalitis in genetically susceptible mice of all ages), we compared NWS growth in A2G aggregates of various developmental stages. The results are shown in Figure 3. In contrast to 32-day-old cultures, undifferentiated 10-day-old A2G cultures allowed viral replication to the same degree as A/J cultures of both ages.

It has been shown that treatment of the whole animal with sheep AIFG abolished inborn resistance to orthomyxoviruses, rendering adult A2G mice fully susceptible to intracerebral infection with NWS virus (*Haller* et al. 1979a). We therefore determined growth of NWS virus in well-differentiated brain cell aggregates of susceptible and resistant genotype in the presence of AIFG or of normal sheep globulin (NSG). To ensure uniform exposure of cells within the aggregates both globulin preparations were added to the cultures 48 h before the virus inoculum and were kept present throughout the experiment. NSG treatment did not change the susceptibility phenotypes of the two types of cultures. AIFG treatment, however, prevented expression of resistance in A2G cultures. It also slightly increased viral growth in genetically susceptible A/J cultures.

It can be concluded that brain cell aggregates behave in vitro with respect to infection with neurotropic influenza virus much like brains of intact animals. In both cases expression of the resistance phenotype is age related and depends on interferon and the host gene *Mx*. These results demonstrate that aggregating brain cell cultures are eminently

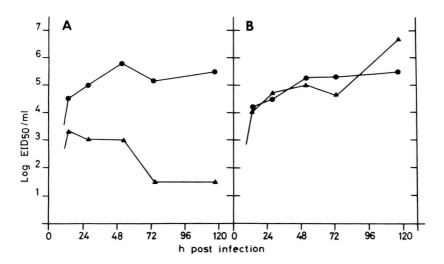

Fig. 3A, B. Age-dependent expression of resistance in aggregating fetal brain cell cultures. Aggregates established from susceptible A/J (●) or resistant A2G mice (▲) were either cultured for 32 days (A) or for 10 days (B) before infection with $10^6$ EID$_{50}$/culture of NWS virus. Cell-free medium from individual cultures was assayed for infectivity at the time indicated. Each point is the mean EID$_{50}$ from two independent cultures. EID$_{50}$, mean egg infective dose

suited for investigations of viral neuropathogenicity and should thus offer a nice approach to the study of virus-host interactions in diseases of the central nervous system.

## 8 The Resistance Gene *Mx* Influences Sensitivity to Interferon Action Selectively for Influenza Virus

We have shown so far that mice bearing the allele *Mx* exhibit a high degree of specific resistance to influenza virus. This resistance is independent of immune defense mechanisms, is expressed in differentiated cells of various organs, and can be abrogated by treatment with potent anti-interferon serum. Thus, peritoneal macrophages taken from *Mx*-bearing animals treated with anti-interferon globulin proved fully susceptible to influenza virus in vitro (*Haller* et al. 1979a). In contrast, freshly cultivated macrophages from untreated resistant mice were resistant even when infected in the presence of AIFG (*Haller* et al. 1979a). We had to pretreat the donor mouse in order to obtain susceptible *Mx*-bearing macrophages. This indicated that, in our conventionally reared animals, peritoneal macrophages were exposed to interferon in vivo. We then observed that this in-vivo-induced resistance of macrophages was gradually lost during prolonged cultivation in vitro in the absence of interferon (*Haller* et al. 1980a, b). After 2–3 weeks in culture, macrophages from resistant animals were phenotypically susceptible to M-TUR virus. We will call these cultured cells "aged" macrophages as opposed to freshly explanted macrophages.

If interferon were responsible for resistance, it should be possible to restore the resistance phenotype of *Mx*-carrying "aged" macrophages by treatment with doses of interferon which would leave non-*Mx*-bearing cells susceptible. Furthermore, it would be necessary to demonstrate virus specificity of interferon action in such cells. In other words, we had to demonstrate that orthomyxoviruses were more sensitive to the antiviral state induced by interferon in *Mx*-bearing cells than in control cells and that the antiviral state toward other viruses was not affected by *Mx*.

### 8.1 Cooperation Between Interferon and the Host Gene *Mx*

Such experiments were performed with cultivated peritoneal macrophages from backcross mice segregating for the two alleles at the *Mx* locus. A2G (*Mx/Mx*) males were mated with C57BL/6 (+/+) females. Backcrosses of the resulting $F_1$ offspring with the susceptible (+/+) parent yielded a first backcross generation (BC-1), 50% of which were *Mx*-carriers as evidenced by resistance of their freshly explanted macrophages. Macrophages from these backcross mice were then cultivated for 3 weeks, at which time their differential sensitivity to graded doses of interferon was determined as indicated in Figure 4.

Figure 5 demonstrates that macrophages kept for 3 weeks in culture were highly susceptible to influenza virus M-TUR irrespective of their genotype. In the absence of interferon, no inhibition of viral replication was detectable, suggesting that no inherent cellular restriction was present in *Mx*-bearing cells. However, pretreatment of these macrophage cultures with as little as 20 reference units per ml of partially purified mouse

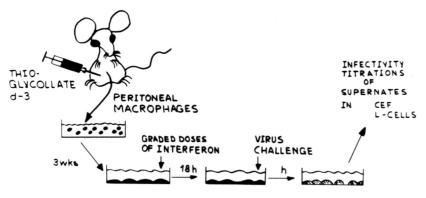

Fig. 4. Test for sensitivity of mouse macrophages to interferon. Thioglycollate-induced peritoneal macrophages obtained from resistant or susceptible animals were cultivated for 3 weeks, at which time they were highly and uniformly susceptible to various test viruses, including macrophage-adapted influenza virus M-TUR. These cultures were then incubated with graded doses of mouse interferon for 18 h before virus challenge. Interferon induced by NDV in mouse C-243 cells purified to either $10^7$ or $10^9$ reference units/mg protein was used (a gift from Drs. *I. Gresser* and *M. Aguet*, Institut de Recherches Scientifiques sur le Cancer, Villejuif, France). Virus yields at various times after infection were determined by infectivity titrations of cell-free medium from individual cultures on chick embryo fibroblast (*CEF*) or L cell monolayers

interferon type I gave an entirely different picture (Figure 6). Interferon treatment caused a slight delay of viral growth in cells lacking the resistance allele. In contrast, the same amount of interferon markedly inhibited viral multiplication in *Mx*-bearing macrophages. These findings indicated that cells carrying the resistance gene were more sensitive to the antiviral action of interferon than cells from genetically susceptible mice when challenged with influenza viruses.

## 8.2 Virus Specificity of Interferon Action

A major difficulty in accepting interferon as an essential element in this form of resistance was the nonspecificity of interferon action. Interferon is said to act against all viruses more or less indiscriminately. It is true that not all viruses are equally sensitive to interferon blockade. When viruses are ranked according to their sensitivity to the antiviral state induced by interferon, their order depends on the animal species used for testing (*Stewart* et al. 1969; *Youngner* et al. 1972). Such a comparison is not very meaningful because two elements are altered, the host tissue and the interferon, which has to be from the homologous species. The allele *Mx* caused resistance only against a narrow spectrum of closely related viruses, the orthomyxoviruses, but not against a large number of other viruses (*Lindenmann* et al. 1963; *Lindenmann* and *Klein* 1966). If interferon was to remain a serious candidate for the mechanism of this resistance, we had to show that the antiviral spectrum of interferon depended on the presence or absence of the allele *Mx*.

Two viruses capable of growing in macrophages, VSV (a rhabdovirus) and EMC (a picornavirus), were therefore compared with M-TUR (influenza A) for reduction of yields by graded doses of interferon in aged *Mx/Mx, Mx/*+ and +/+ macrophages. Figure

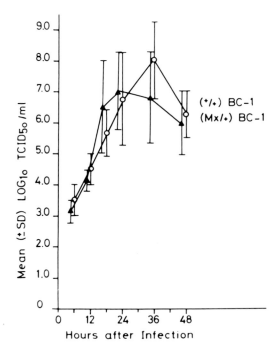

Fig. 5. Growth of M-TUR virus in aged macrophage cultures from backcross mice segregating for the allele *Mx*. After 3 weeks in culture, peritoneal macrophages obtained from individual *Mx/*+ or +/+ backcross mice (*BC-I*) were infected with M-TUR virus at a multiplicity of 5. After incubation for 90 min at 37 °C the virus inoculum was removed by repeated washings. Cell-free medium from individual cultures was titrated on primary chick embryo fibroblast monolayers at the times indicated. Titers represent mean values from three macrophage cultures of either resistant *Mx/*+ (▲) or susceptible +/+ (O) genotype

7 shows that whereas yields of VSV and EMC were similarly inhibited in all types of cells, yields of M-TUR were markedly reduced in homozygous (*Mx/Mx*) and heterozygous (*Mx/*+) cells from resistant animals but much less reduced in cells from susceptible (+/+) mice. Yields of M-TUR virus in macrophages not pretreated with interferon were not influenced by the presence or absence of the host resistance gene *Mx*.

To exclude the possibility that this resistance phenomenon was a peculiarity of macrophages, it had to be reproduced in other cell types as well. Since we had at our disposal an influenza virus strain highly pathogenic for mouse liver and since adult rat and mouse hepatocytes in primary monolayer cultures were known to preserve specialized cell functions in vitro (*Berry* and *Friend* 1969; *Renton* et al. 1978), virus susceptibility of hepatocytes from resistant and susceptible adult mice was tested.

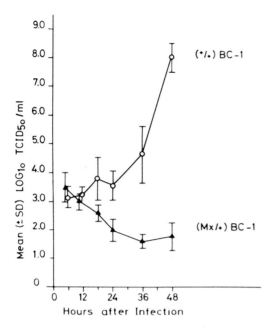

Fig. 6. Inhibition by interferon of multiplication of M-TUR virus in macrophage cultures from backcross mice BC-1 segregating for the allele *Mx*. After 3 weeks in culture, peritoneal macrophages obtained from individual *Mx*/+ or +/+ backcross mice were incubated for 18 h with 20 reference units of mouse interferon induced by NDV in mouse C-243 cells and partially purified to $1 \times 10^7$ reference units/mg protein. Cells were then washed and infected with M-TUR virus at a multiplicity of 5. After incubation for 30 min at 37 °C the virus inoculum was removed by repeated washings. Cell-free medium from individual cultures was titrated on primary chick embryo fibroblast monolayers at the times after infection indicated. Titers represent mean values from three macrophage cultures of either resistance *Mx*/+ (▲) or susceptible +/+ genotype (○). $TCID_{50}$, mean tissue culture infective dose

## 8.3 *Mx* Gene Expression in Monolayer Cultures of Adult Hepatocytes

Primary monolayer cultures of adult mouse hepatocytes isolated by enzymatic perfusion of the liver in situ were prepared by a modification of the method originally described by *Berry* and *Friend* (1969). Adult mouse hepatocytes in culture represent a homogenous population of cells which are nonproliferating, are well differentiated, and maintain regulatory cell functions in vitro (*Bissell* 1976; *Bonney* et al. 1974). Such cultures were found to be suited for the study of productive infection with a variety of hepatotropic viruses (*Arnheiter* 1980). Both the hepatotropic influenza virus strain TURH and the macrophage-adapted variant M-TUR originally derived from TURH (*Lindenmann* et al. 1978) showed high pathogenicity for hepatocytes isolated from genetically susceptible mice. With a large challenge dose, maximum release of infectious virus and hemagglutinin occurred simultaneously with total monolayer destruction 24 h after infection.

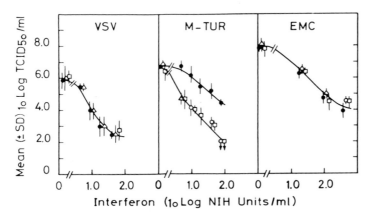

Fig. 7. Effects of interferon on multiplication of VSV, M-TUR and EMC virus in macrophages from resistant or susceptible mice. Peritoneal macrophages from resistant mice homozygous (□) or heterozygous (△) for the allele *Mx*, and from susceptible +/+ mice (●) were cultured for 3 weeks and were then incubated for 18 h with various doses of partially purified mouse interferon. Thereafter, cultures were washed and infected at a multiplicity of 5 with either VSV, M-TUR, or EMC virus. After an incubation period of 60 min at 37 °C the virus inoculum was removed by repeated washings. The viral titer of cell-free medium from three individual cultures per interferon dilution was determined 18 h after viral infection (at the time of peak virus production in control cultures). VSV and EMC virus was titered in monolayer cultures of L cells and M-TUR virus in CEF. Mean $TCID_{50}$ values and standard deviations are indicated. The differences in yields of M-TUR virus between interferon-treated +/+ and *Mx*-bearing macrophage cultures were statistically significant ($P < 0.01$ for all interferon doses used)

In contrast, A2G hepatocytes cultured for 24 h resisted infection with either TURH or M-TUR virus. Resistance of *Mx*-bearing liver cells was evidenced by a 100-fold lower maximal infectivity of culture supernates and by absence of monolayer destruction (Fig. 8). However, when A2G cultures were infected at high multiplicities 2 h after cell plating, they were equally permissive for influenza virus replication as A/J cultures (*Arnheiter* et al. 1980). When supernatant fluids of uninfected A/J and A2G hepatocyte cultures were tested for presence of interferon, titers equivalent to 320 reference units per ml were detected in both types of cultures 12 h after cell plating. The antiviral activity observed seemed to be of interferon type I, since it could be neutralized by antibodies against type I interferon and shared some physicochemical properties with this type of interferon (*Arnheiter* et al. 1980). The mechanisms leading to spontaneous interferon release in hepatocyte cultures are at present unknown. Consequently, the development of antiviral resistance in *Mx*-bearing hepatocytes could be prevented by addition of anti-interferon serum. The resistance phenotype could be restored with highly purified interferon, indicating that it was indeed interferon and not some other antivirally active constituent which acted in conjunction with the resistance gene. Thus, hepatocytes from adult animals behaved essentially the same as peritoneal macrophages: The antiviral state created with the help of endogenous or exogenous interferon was much more active on influenza virus in cells bearing the allele *Mx* than in cells lacking it.

In order to confirm the specificity of antiviral protection realized by cooperation of interferon with the host gene *Mx*, the degree of interferon-induced resistance against

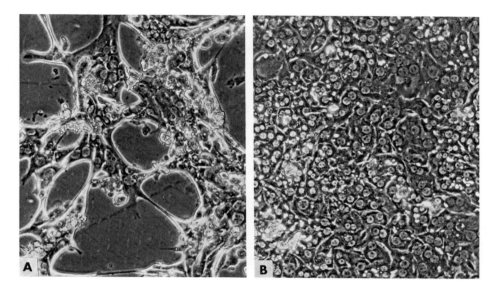

Fig. 8. Cytopathic effect produced by influenza A virus in hepatocyte cultures derived from suscept-ible A/J or resistant A2G mice. Hepatocytes were cultured for 24 h before infection with M-TUR at a multiplicity of 10. A/J monolayers were destroyed 24 h after infection (A), whereas A2G monolayers retained their integrity (B). Magnification 200×

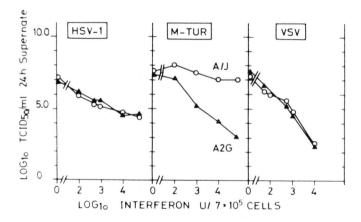

Fig. 9. Antiviral protection of A/J and A2G hepatocyte cultures by exogenous interferon. Establish-ment of an antiviral state by spontaneously liberated interferon was prevented by addition of anti-interferon antibodies from 0 to 24 h after cell isolation. Cultures were then washed four times and exposed to graded doses of partially purified type I interferon or to control medium for 18 h. The cul-tures were washed again and infected with herpes simplex virus type 1 (*HSV-I*) at a multiplicity of 0.1, influenza virus M-TUR at a multiplicity of 10, or vesicular stomatitis virus (*VSV*) at a multiplicity of 10. Infectivity was assayed 24 h after infection. Values are given as mean from two independent cul-tures. O–O A/J cultures; ▲-▲, A2G cultures

infection with three unrelated viruses was assessed. The challenge viruses were Herpes simplex virus type 1 (HSV-1), a DNA virus, and two RNA viruses, influenza virus M-TUR and vesicular stomatitis virus (VSV). Figure 9 shows the comparison of 24-h yields of these viruses in A2G (*Mx/Mx*) and A/J (+/+) hepatocytes treated with graded doses of partially purified mouse interferon. Untreated *Mx/Mx* hepatocytes were equally permissive for all three viruses as +/+ hepatocytes. However, increasing amounts of interferon impeded the growth of M-TUR virus in *Mx*-bearing hepatocytes, but hardly affected the same virus in +/+ control cells. By contrast, interferon had the same inhibitory power against HSV-1 in both *Mx*-carrying cells and in controls. Similarly, inhibition of VSV multiplication was independent of the host cell genotype. Thus, in hepatocytes homozygous for *Mx*, M-TUR behaved as if it were a virus highly sensitive to interferon action (in fact, as sensitive as VSV), whereas in +/+ cells it behaved as a virus extremely insensitive to interferon (being the least sensitive of the three viruses tested).

These results indicated that virus-specific enhanced sensitivity to interferon was most likely a property of all adult A2G cells. Interestingly, larger amounts of interferon were required for antiviral protection of hepatocytes as compared to macrophages. Preliminary results indicate that mouse kidney cells could hardly be protected, even with huge doses of interferon, whatever their genotype. These differences in interferon sensitivity between various cell types may in part explain the initial failure to detect expression of resistance in tissue culture. Whether the age-related expression of the resistance phenotype observed in aggregating brain cell cultures was due to an increase in interferon sensitivity or an increase in interferon production is not known at present.

## 8.4 Kinetics of the Antiviral State Induced by Interferon in Cells Bearing *Mx*

After exposure to interferon, cells require several hours of incubation for full expression of antiviral activity. The antiviral state, once developed, is maintained for a certain period of time after which cells return to their previous virus-sensitive condition. Thus, a rise and fall of interferon-induced antiviral activity can be described (*Stewart* 1979). To elucidate the interaction between *Mx* and interferon we have studied the kinetics of the interferon-induced antiviral activity in *Mx*-bearing and non-*Mx*-bearing macrophages.

In a first experiment the development of the antiviral state was investigated. Aged macrophages were treated with mouse interferon for defined periods of time before infection with either influenza virus M-TUR or VSV. Figure 10 shows that the antiviral state toward M-TUR developed much faster and to higher levels in cells carrying the resistance gene *Mx* than in cells lacking *Mx*. This was true even when the latter were exposed to 250 times higher interferon concentrations than *Mx*-bearing macrophages (Fig. 10a). In contrast, antiviral activity to VSV developed equally well and to the same degree in cells of both genotypes (Fig. 10b). In conclusion, whereas the allele *Mx* enhanced the development of the antiviral potential toward influenza virus, it did not influence the development of the antiviral state toward VSV.

We then analyzed the duration of the antiviral state in aged macrophages of susceptible or resistant genotype against M-TUR or VSV. Again, the allele *Mx* was found to influence the rate of decay of interferon-induced resistance in a virus-specific way as demonstrated in Figure 11. It can be seen that A2G cells treated for 18 h with minute concentrations of interferon (4–40 reference units/ml) remained in a virus-resistant state for

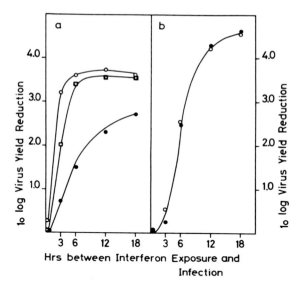

Fig. 10a, b. Development of the antiviral state to M-TUR or VSV in macrophages of resistant or susceptible genotype. "Aged" macrophages from A2G (*open symbols*) or A/J mice (*closed symbols*) were treated with partially purified mouse interferon type I ($10^7$ reference units/mg protein) for the periods of time indicated. Treated cells were then washed and were infected together with untreated control cells in the presence of AIFG (neutralizing capacity of $10^4$ reference units of interferon). Virus inocula consisted of influenza virus M-TUR (a) at a multiplicity of 10 and of VSV (b) at a multiplicity of 10. Interferon concentrations used to protect cells against M-TUR (a) were 40 (□) and $10^4$ (○, ●) reference units/ml. Forty reference units/ml were used to protect cells against VSV (b). Virus yields were determined 18 h after infection (at the time of peak virus production in control cultures), and virus yield reduction was calculated as $Log_{10}$ (yields in untreated control cultures/yields in interferon-treated cultures)

many days when the challenge virus was M-TUR (Fig. 11a). On the other hand, A/J cells treated with $10^4$ reference units/ml regained full virus susceptibility within 4 days (Fig. 11b). However, the decay rate of the antiviral state against VSV was exactly the same in A/J and A2G cultures (Fig. 11c). It should be noted that in these experiments true decay rates were measured because residual interferon activity was neutralized by anti-interferon antibody added to the cultures after interferon removal.

These experiments have revealed great differences in development and duration of the antiviral state to influenza virus (but not VSV) between cells bearing *Mx* and those devoid of it. Trivial explanations such as differences in interferon receptors seemed most unlikely in view of the virus specificity of the phenomenon. It seemed possible, however, that inhibition at the molecular level would present distinctive features.

## 8.5 Influenza Virus Replication is Inhibited at an Early Step

We have therefore performed polyacrylamide gel electrophoresis of viral proteins in aged macrophages from either resistant (*Mx/Mx*) or susceptible (+/+) mice with or

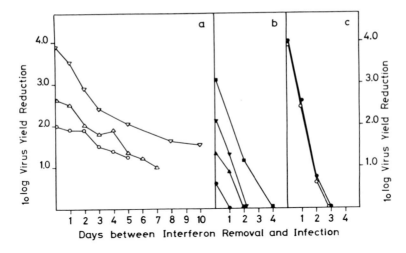

Fig. 11a–c. Decay of antiviral state to M-TUR or VSV in macrophages of resistant or susceptible genotype. "Aged" macrophages from A2G (*open symbols*) or A/J mice (*closed symbols*) were treated for 18 h with partially purified mouse interferon type I ($10^7$ reference units/mg protein). Treated cells were then washed and were further incubated in the presence of AIFG (at concentrations sufficient to neutralize $10^4$ reference units of interferon) for the periods of time indicated before infection with M-TUR (a, b) or VSV (c) at multiplicities of 10. Interferon concentrations used to protect A2G cells against M-TUR (a) were 4 (○), 10 (△) and 40 (▽) reference units/ml. Interferon concentrations used to protect A/J cells against M-TUR b were 40 (●), 400 (▲), $10^3$ (▼) and $10^4$ (■) reference units/ml. Forty reference units/ml were used to protect cells against VSV (c). $Log_{10}$ virus yield reduction was determined as in Fig. 10

without pretreatment with interferon (*Horisberger* et al. 1980). Anti-interferon serum was added at the time of infection, so that only the amount of interferon used to pretreat the cells influenced the results shown in Figure 12. Synthesis of viral proteins was obvious in both types of macrophages in the absence of interferon (lanes 7 and 10); addition of anti-interferon serum at the time of infection did not alter virus protein patterns (lanes 8 and 11). Pretreatment with 40 reference units of interferon, followed by anti-interferon serum, greatly inhibited viral protein synthesis in *Mx/Mx* macrophages (lane 9), but had no measurable effect on that in +/+ macrophages (lane 12). This gel pattern represents protein synthesis 7 h after infection. All identifiable proteins appear to be similarly inhibited.

A comparable picture was obtained with freshly explanted macrophages. In fresh susceptible (+/+) macrophages newly formed virus-specific proteins were readily detectable 7 h after infection, whereas viral protein synthesis was virtually absent in fresh macrophages from resistant (*Mx/Mx*) animals.

It was conceivable that the observed differences in virus replication were due to differences in virus attachment or penetration. Differences in viral receptors on pancreatic beta cells, for instance, have been implicated in the ability of EMC virus to cause diabetes mellitus in various strains of mice (*Chairez* et al. 1978). However, no differences in viral attachment between resistant and susceptible macrophages could be revealed by two independent methods measuring either radioactivity or infectivity of the virus input. Similarly, virus penetration seemed not to be affected (*Horisberger* et al. 1980).

CONTROL      INFECTED

Genotype  Mx/Mx    +/+     Mx/Mx    +/+
IF units  − − 40 −  − − 40 − − 40 −  − − 40
          1  2  3  4  5  6  7  8  9 10 11 12

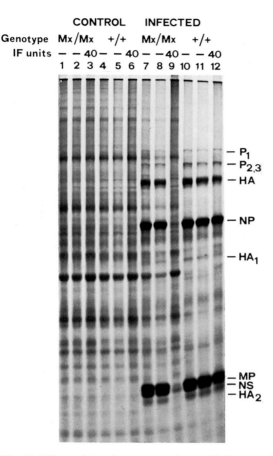

— P₁
— P₂,₃
— HA

— NP

— HA₁

— MP
— NS
— HA₂

Fig. 12. Effects of interferon on synthesis of influenza virus proteins in aged macrophages from resistant A2G (*Mx/Mx*) or susceptible A/J (+/+) mice. Peritoneal macrophages from mice genetically *Mx/Mx* (lanes 1–3 and 7–9) or +/+ (lanes 4–6 and 10–12) were kept for 3 weeks in culture and were then incubated for 18 h with either 40 reference units/ml of partially purified mouse interferon (lanes 3, 6, 9, 12) or normal control medium. Interferon pretreated and untreated cells were washed and infected with M-TUR virus at multiplicities of 5 (lanes 7–12). Sheep anti-mouse interferon globulin diluted to give a neutralizing titer of $1.2 \times 10^{-3}$ was added at the time of infection to all but four culture wells to which normal sheep globulin was added (lanes 1, 4, 7, 10). Infected and uninfected control cells were labeled for 30 min with $^{35}$S-methionine at 7 h after infection. Whole-cell lysates were prepared and were subjected to electrophoresis on 11% polyacrylamide slab gels as described by *Horisberger* et al. 1980; *Laemmli* and *Favre* 1973. Autoradiography revealed the following viral proteins: polymerase-associated polypeptides ($P_1$, $P_{2, 3}$), uncleaved hemagglutinin *(HA)* and hemagglutinin cleavage products (HA₁, *HA₂*), nucleoprotein *(NP)*, matrix protein *(MP)*, and non-structural proteins *(NS)*

The present data show that the block caused by the gene *Mx* together with interferon occurs at an early stage in influenza virus replication and that it must be localized somewhere between virus penetration and transcription or translation. Viral protein and RNA synthesis are so interdependent that it is difficult to analyze which of the two might be predominantly affected; both have also been implicated in the antiviral action of interferon against influenza virus in cells not carrying the gene *Mx* (*Bean* and *Simpson* 1973; *Repik* et al. 1974). Future investigations on viral uncoating, primary transcription, and translation should help to clarify the very step at which interferon, together with the host gene *Mx,* can realize an antiviral state exhibiting considerable specificity for a group of closely related viruses.

## 9 Genetic Control of Interferon Action in Vivo

It is evident that these results showing a genetic control of sensitivity to interferon action specific for a given virus in vitro are related to the in vivo resistance of A2G mice to influenza virus. Interferon levels in brains and sera of adult A2G mice resisting influenza virus infection were constantly found to be much lower than those of susceptible A/J mice dying from infection (*Fiske* and *Klein* 1975; *Haller* et al. 1979a). In vivo resistance was presumably not due to greater production of interferon during infection but to greater sensitivity to interferon action. Interferon formed during the first cycles of virus replication was probably very efficient in inhibiting influenza virus spread in various organs in the presence of *Mx*, whereas it was inefficient in the absence of *Mx*. When interferon was neutralized by specific antibody, *Mx*-gene-controlled resistance was no longer detectable.

Treatment with anti-interferon serum has been so far the only means of rendering resistant mice susceptible to influenza virus. There are, however, two other instances in which inborn resistance of *Mx* carriers is not manifested. As in most cases of genetic resistance of mice to viral infections, newborn animals are fully susceptible (*Lindenmann* 1964; *Hirsch* et al. 1970; *Sabin* 1952; *Gallily* et al. 1967; *Neighbour* et al. 1978). Furthermore, exceptional influenza virus strains have been detected which are lethal for normal adult A2G mice (*Lindenmann* et al. 1963; *Lindenmann* and *Klein* 1966). There are, of course, many possibilities to account for these observations of genuine A2G susceptibility. One possibility is inadequate interferon production during infection. In this case treatment with interferon should be protective and should allow one to detect possible genetic differences between strains of mice in interferon sensitivity in vivo.

## 9.1 Protection of Newborn Mice by Exogenous Interferon

In *Mx* heterozygotes resistance to hepatotropic influenza virus TURH is not fully established before 2 weeks of age (unpublished observations). Since disease develops extremely fast and culminates in death on day 2 to 3 after lethal infection, we decided to test the protective effect of exogenous interferon against TURH infection in *Mx*-bearing and non-*Mx*-bearing newborns. (A2G × CBA/J)F$_1$ (genetically *Mx*/+) and (A/J × CBA/J) F$_1$ (genetically +/+) newborn mice were injected subcutaneously in the interscapular region with partially purified mouse interferon type I daily for the first 3 days of birth. Each mouse received a total amount of $8 \times 10^5$ reference units of interferon. Controls within the same litter were inoculated with a mock interferon preparation. All animals were infected on day 2 with 100 LD$_{50}$ of TURH virus given intraperitoneally. Table 5 shows that all control *Mx*-bearing mice died at the same time as their +/+ counterparts. Interferon treatment somewhat delayed but did not prevent death in (A/J × CBA/J)F$_1$

Table 5. Protection of newborn mice against lethal influenza virus infection by interferon[a]

| Newborn animals | | Controls | | Interferon treated | |
|---|---|---|---|---|---|
| Strain | Genotype | No. surviving 3 wks/total No. injected | Mean day of death | No. surviving 3 wks/total No. injected | Mean day of death |
| (A/J x CBA/J)F$_1$ | +/+ | 0/19 | 2.5 | 0/20 | 3.2 |
| (A2G x CBA/J)F$_1$ | Mx/+ | 0/14 | 2.5 | 16/16 | – |

[a] Newborn mice were injected subcutaneously in the interscapular region with partially purified mouse interferon type I (induced by NDV in mouse C-243 cells and containing $10^7$ reference units/mg protein) on day 1, day 2, and day 3 to a total amount of $8 \times 10^5$ reference units per mouse. Controls within the same litter were inoculated with a mock interferon preparation. Animals were infected intraperitoneally on day 2 with 100 LD$_{50}$ of hepatotropic influenza virus TURH

animals. In contrast, all 16 (A2G × CBA/J)F$_1$ hybrid mice inoculated survived infection for more than 3 weeks without signs of disease. These results clearly showed that a given amount of interferon rendered Mx carriers resistant to influenza virus, whereas the same amount was insufficient to protect mice devoid of Mx against the same virus challenge. These results were in complete agreement with our findings on phenotype expression in hepatocytes in vitro.

## 9.2 Protection of Adult Mx-Bearing Mice against an A2G-Virulent Influenza Virus Strain by Interferon Inducers

Since the discovery of A2G resistance by *Lindenmann* in 1962 (*Lindenmann* 1962), a large number of influenza virus strains have been tested for mouse pathogenicity, and all but a few strains have been found to be less virulent for A2G than for control mice. Resistance was operative against virus strains of the most diverse origins and passage histories (*Lindenmann* and *Klein* 1966). Two Asian influenza A2 strains derived from one of the earliest isolates, A2/Singapore/1/57, were lethal for A2G mice (*Lindenmann* et al. 1963). We have recently observed that a human influenza A strain isolated in our laboratory many years ago and identified as PR8 was equally pathogenic for A2G and control mice.

These A2G-virulent influenza virus strains might be considered as mutants able to overcome the resistance barrier established by Mx and interferon. Alternatively, these viruses might be equally sensitive to the resistance mechanism but might fail to induce it, most likely because of an inability to induce sufficient amounts of interferon.

To test whether our A2G-virulent PR8 strain was restricted by the antiviral state induced by interferon in the presence of the resistance gene Mx, we pretreated A2G and control mice with various interferon inducers before infection. Newcastle disease virus (NDV) is among the best inducers of interferon in the mouse (*Baron* and *Buckler* 1963). Circulating interferon produced in mice after inoculation with NDV is under control of a single autosomal locus, designated *If-1* (*De Maeyer* and *De Maeyer-Guignard* 1969). Two alleles have been described, *If-1$^h$* for high and *If-1$^l$* for low interferon responsiveness (*De Maeyer* et al. 1970). The *If-1* locus has a quantitative rather than a qualitative effect on serum interferon levels in response to NDV (*Bailey* and *De Maeyer-Guignard* 1972). *If-1* control of interferon production is specific for NDV. Additional *If* loci have been reported segregating independently from *If-1*, each of which determines interferon production to a particular virus (*De Maeyer* et al. 1974). A2G mice are *If-1$^h$* (*Mouse News Letter* 1977). We therefore injected A2G and control mice homozygous for *If-1$^h$* with NDV 24 h before intranasal infection with 5000 lethal doses (as measured in untreated A2G mice) of A2G-virulent PR8 virus. NDV pretreatment resulted in equal serum interferon titers in both strains of mice. A2G mice were protected, whereas non-*Mx*-bearing controls succumbed to infection (Experiment 1, Table 6).

In a second experiment, high molecular weight double-stranded polyribonucleotides, i.e. polyriboinosinic-polyribocytidylic acid (poly I:C), were used as inducers of interferon (*Torrence* and *De Clercq* 1977; *Field* et al. 1967). Although interferon levels 2 h after induction were highest in the non-*Mx*-carriers, these were not protected. Again, inducer-pretreated but not untreated A2G mice were resistant and survived (Table 6). Comparable results were obtained with a third interferon inducer, the low molecular weight substance tilorone (data not shown).

## 10 Concluding Remarks

We have presented here current evidence for a genetic control of sensitivity to interferon action at the single cell level resulting in virus-specific host resistance. It is of interest that a similar concept has also been discussed with regard to flaviviruses (*Hanson* et al. 1969). Hanson and collaborators have found that cultures of cells from mice genetically resistant to flaviviruses are much more susceptible to the inhibitory effect of mouse interferon when tested with flaviviruses than cultures from susceptible mice (*Hanson* et al. 1969).

Table 6. Effect of interferon inducers on pathogenicity of A2G-virulent strain of influenza virus PR8[a]

| Exp. | Interferon inducer | Mouse strain and genotype | | Serum interferon units/ml | No. surviving 3 wks/total No. injected | Mean day of death |
|---|---|---|---|---|---|---|
| 1 | NDV | C57BL/6J | (+/+) | 400 | 0/7 | 6.3 |
| | NDV | A2G | (*Mx/Mx*) | 400 | 7/7 | – |
| | none | C57BL/6J | (+/+) | 0 | 0/7 | 5.4 |
| | none | A2G | (*Mx/Mx*) | 0 | 0/7 | 5.8 |
| 2 | Poly I:C | CBA/J | (+/+) | 3200 | 1/5 | 5.5 |
| | Poly I:C | A/J | (+/+) | 1600 | 0/5 | 5.2 |
| | Poly I:C | A2G | (*Mx/Mx*) | 600 | 5/5 | – |
| | none | CBA/J | (+/+) | 0 | 0/5 | 6.2 |
| | none | A/J | (+/+) | 0 | 0/5 | 4.6 |
| | none | A2G | (*Mx/Mx*) | 0 | 0/5 | 5.8 |

[a] NDV ($10^8$ $EID_{50}$/mouse, i.v.) or Poly I:C (50 µg/mouse, i.p.) were injected 24 h before infection with 5000 $LD_{50}$ (exp. 1) or 50 $LD_{50}$ (exp. 2) of A2G-virulent PR8 virus intranasally. Controls received saline i.v. or i.p. Sera were collected 18 h (exp. 1) or 2 h (exp. 2) after inoculation of the inducer. Sera were pooled per group, treated at low pH, and assayed for interferon activity on mouse L cells infected with VSV. C57BL/6 J and A2G are both genetically *If-1 h/h*

Moreover, interferon appears to be a key factor in inborn resistance of mice to mouse hepatitis virus (*Virelizier* and *Gresser* 1978) and to herpes simplex virus (*Zawatzky* et al. 1979).

The *Mx* gene system may therefore be but one example of a whole family of resistance genes operating via interferon mechanisms. Hypotheses on the details of the interaction between *Mx* and interferon remain speculative. Cooperation between the host gene *Mx* and interferon results in the establishment of an antiviral state which is particularly efficient in inhibiting orthomyxoviruses. We could explain this by assuming that essentially one antiviral state is created but that its shape (the extent to which it affects the biosynthetic demands of various viruses) is host gene dependent. Or we could envisage the overal antiviral state as being composed of several discrete antiviral sectors, each specialized in inhibiting one particular group of viruses.

A prominent character of the interferon system has been its lack of virus specificity. Nevertheless, it would now appear that in the mouse a certain degree of specificity may occur both at the level of interferon production and at the level of interferon action. Thus, inbred mouse strains are known to differ significantly in their ability to produce interferon in response to a given virus. Several *If* loci have been found to control the amount of circulating interferon which is produced after injection of mice with different viruses (*De Maeyer* and *De Maeyer-Guignard* 1969; *De Maeyer* et al. 1974). Here we have presented evidence for host gene control of sensitivity to interferon action selectively for a particular group of viruses.

If applicable to man, the present result might provide a clue to the better understanding of individual variations in susceptibility to viral diseases. It is conceivable that similar interactions between interferon and host genes could be important not only in pathogenesis of viral infections but also with respect to nonantiviral effects of interferon. In fact, differences in the immunomodulatory effects of type I interferon according to genotype have recently been described (*De Maeyer* and *De Maeyer-Guignard* 1980). New technology and mass production will soon allow a broad clinical application of human interferons. Genetic control of interferon action may be more general than has hitherto been supposed and should be considered in clinical trials.

*Acknowledgments.* I thank Drs. *Heinz Arnheiter, Michel Horisberger,* and *Jean Lindenmann* for contributions to and critical review of the manuscript, Mrs. *Martha Acklin* and Mr. *Gerold Barmettler* for technical assistance, and Mrs. *Ruth Leemann* for preparing the manuscript. Research described in this review is supported by grants no. 3.139–0.77 and 3.393–0.78 from the Swiss National Science Foundation.

# References

Allison AC (1974) Interactions of antibodies, complement components and various cell types in immunity against viruses and pyogenic bacteria. Transplant Rev 19:3

Aguet M (1980) Specific binding of [125]I labelled purified and biologically acitve mouse interferon to mouse leukemia L 1210 and L 929 cells. Nature 284:459

Arnheiter H (1980) Primary monolayer culture of adult mouse hepatocytes: a model for the study of hepatotropic viruses. Arch Virol 63:11

Arnheiter H, Haller O, Lindenmann J (1980) Host gene influence on interferon action in adult mouse hepatocytes: specificity for influenza virus. Virology 103:11

Bailey MD, De Maeyer-Guignard J (1972) Molecular weight of serum interferon induced by the Newcastle disease virus in high and low producer mice. Ann Inst Pasteur (Paris) 123:835

Balner H (1963) Identification of peritoneal macrophages in mouse radiation chimeras. Transplantation 1:217

Bang FB (1978) Genetics of resistance of animals to viruses: I. Introduction and studies in mice. Adv Virus Res 23:269

Bang FB, Warwick A (1960) Mouse macrophages as host cells for the mouse hepatitis virus and the genetic basis of their susceptibility. Proc Natl Acad Sci USA 46:1065

Baron S, Buckler CE (1963) Circulating interferon in mice after intravenous injection of virus. Science 141:1061

Bean WJ, Simpson RW (1973) Primary transcription of the influenza virus genome is permissive cells. Virology 56:646

Bennett M (1973) Prevention of marrow allograft rejection with radioactive strontium: evidence for marrow-dependent effector cells. J Immunol 110:510

Berry MN, Friend DS (1969) High-yield preparation of isolated rat liver parenchymal cells: a biochemical and fine structural study. J Cell Biol 43:506

Bissell DM (1976) Study of hepatocyte function in cell culture. Prog Liver Dis 5:69

Bonney RJ, Becker JE, Walker PR, Potter VR (1974) Primary monolayer cultures of adult rat liver parenchymal cells suitable for study of the regulation of enzyme synthesis. In Vitro 9:399

Chairez R, Yoon JW, Notkins AL (1978) Virus-induced diabetes mellitus. X. Attachment of encephalo-myocarditis virus and permissiveness of cultures pancreatic β cells to infection. Virology 85:606

Crofton RW, Diesselhoff-den Dulk MM, Furth R van (1978) The origin, kinetics, and characteristics of the Kupffer cells in the normal steady state. J Exp Med 148:1

De Maeyer E, De Maeyer-Guignard J (1969) Gene with quantitative effect on circulating interferon induced by Newcastle disease virus. J Virol 3:506

De Maeyer E, De Maeyer-Guignard J (1980) Host genotype influences immunomodulation by interferon. Nature 284:173

De Maeyer E, De Maeyer-Guignard J, Jullien P (1970) Circulating interferon production in the mouse: origin and nature of cells involved and influence of animal genotype. J Gen Physiol 56:435

De Maeyer E, De Maeyer-Guignard J, Hall WT, Bailey DW (1974) A locus affecting circulating interferon levels induced by mouse mammary tumor virus. J Gen Virol 23:209

Fauconnier B (1970) Augmentation de la pathogénicité virale par l'emploi de sérum anti-interferon in vivo. CR Acad Sci [D] (Paris) 271:464

Field TK, Tytell AA, Lampson GP, Hilleman MR (1967) Inducers of interferon and host resistance. II. Multistranded synthetic polynucleotide complexes. Proc Natl Acad Sci USA 58:1004

Fiske RA, Klein PA (1975) Effect of immunosuppression on the genetic resistance of A2G mice to neurovirulent influenza virus. Infect Immun 11:576

Gale RP, Sparkes RS, Golde DW (1978) Bone marrow origin of hepatic macrophages (Kupffer cells) in humans. Science 201:937

Galliliy R, Warwick A, Bang FB (1967) Ontogeny of macrophage resistance to mouse hepatitis in vivo and in vitro. J Exp Med 125:537

Godleski JJ, Brain JD (1972) The origin of alveolar macrophages in mouse radiation chimeras. J Exp Med 136:630

Goodman GT, Koprowski H (1961) Macrophages as the cellular expression of inherited natural resistance. Proc Natl Acad Sci USA 48:160

Gresser I, Tovey MG, Bandu MT, Maury C, Brouty-Boyé D (1976a) Role of interferon in the pathogenesis of virus diseases in mice as demonstrated by the use of antiinterferon serum. I. Rapid evolution of encephalomyocarditis virus infection. J Exp Med 144:1305

Gresser I, Tovey MG, Maury C, Bandu MT (1976b) Role of interferon in the pathogenesis of virus diseases in mice as demonstrated by the use of anti-interferon serum. II. Studies with herpes simplex, Moloney sarcoma, vesicular stomatitis, Newcastle disease, and influenza viruses. J Exp Med 144:1316

Haller O (1975) A mouse hepatotropic variant of influenza virus. Arch Virol 49:99

Haller O, Honegger P (to be published) Interferon dependent genetic resistance to neuropathogenic influenza virus: aggregating fetal mouse brain cells as a differentiation model

Haller O, Lindenmann J (1974) Athymic (nude) mice express gene for myxovirus resistance. Nature 250:679

Haller O, Wigzell H (1977) Suppression of natural killer cell activity with radioactive strontium: effector cells are marrow-dependent. J Immunol 118:1503

Haller O, Arnheiter H, Lindenmann J (1976) Genetically determined resistance to infection by hepatotropic influenza A virus in mice: effect of immunosuppression. Infect Immun 13:844

Haller O, Kiessling R, Örn A, Wigzell H (1977a) Generation of natural killer cells: an autonomous function of the bone marrow. J Exp Med 145:1411

Haller O, Hansson M, Kiessling R, Wigzell H (1977b) Role of non-conventional natural killer cells in resistance against syngeneic tumour cells in vivo. Nature 270:609

Haller O, Arnheiter H, Gresser IL, Lindenmann J (1979a) Genetically determined, interferon-dependent resistance to influenza virus in mice. J Exp Med 149:601

Haller O, Arnheiter H, Lindenmann J (1979b) Natural, genetically determined resistance toward influenza virus in hemopoietic mouse chimeras. Role of mononuclear phagocytes. J Exp Med 150:117

Haller O, Arnheiter H, Lindenmann J, Gresser I (1980a) In: De Weck E (ed) Biochemical characterization of lymphokines. Proceedings of the Second International Lymphokine Workshop, Ermatingen, Switzerland. Academic Press, New York, pp 393–396

Haller O, Arnheiter H, Lindenmann J, Gresser I (1980b) Host gene influences sensitivity to interferon action selectively for influenza virus. Nature 283:660

Hanson B, Koprowski H, Baron S, Buckler CE (1969) Interferon-mediated natural resistance of mice to arbo B virus infection. Microbios 1B:51

Herberman RB, Holden HT (1978) Natural cell mediated immunity. Adv Cancer Res 27:305

Hirsch MS, Zisman B, Allison AC (1970) Macrophages and age-dependent resistance to herpes simplex virus in mice. J Immunol 104:1160

Honegger P, Richelson E (1976) Biochemical differentiation of mechanically dissociated mammalian brain in aggregating cell culture. Brain Res 109:335

Honegger P, Lenoir D, Favrod P (1979) Growth and differentiation of aggregating fetal brain cells in a serum-free defined medium. Nature 282:305

Horisberger MA, Haller O, Arnheiter H (1980) Interferon-dependent, genetic resistance to influenza virus in mice: viral replication in macrophages is inhibited at an early step. J Gen Virol 50:205

Howard JG (1970) The origin and immunological significance of Kupffer cells. In: Furth R van (ed) Mononuclear phagocytes. Blackwell, Oxford, pp 178

Isaacs A, Hitchcock G (1960) Role of interferon in recovery from virus infections. Lancet 2:69

Johnson RT (1964) The pathogenesis of herpes virus encephalitis. II. A cellular basis for the development of resistance with age. J Exp Med 120:359

Kiessling R, Haller O (1978) Natural killer cells in the mouse: an alternative immune surveillance mechanism? In: Warner NL, Cooper MD (eds) Contemporary topics in immunobiology. Plenum, New York, pp 171–201

Klein J (1975) Biology of the mouse histocompatibility-2 complex. Springer, Berlin Heidelberg New York, p 120

Kumar V, Bennett M, Eckner RJ (1974) Mechanisms of genetic resistance to Friend virus leukemia in mice. I. Role of $^{89}$Sr-sensitive effector cells responsible for rejection of bone marrow allografts. J Exp Med 139:1093

Laemmli UK, Favre M (1973) Maturation of the head of bacteriophage T4. I. DNA packaging events. J Mol Biol 80:575

Lindenmann J (1962) Resistance of mice to mouse-adapted influenza A virus. Virology 16:203

Lindenmann J (1964) Inheritance of resistance to influenza virus in mice. Proc Soc Exp Biol Med 116:506

Lindenmann J, Klein PA (1966) Further studies on the resistance of mice to myxoviruses. Arch Gesamte Virusforsch 19:1

Lindenmann J, Lance CA, Hobson D (1963) The resistance of A2G mice to myxoviruses. J Immunol 90:942

Lindenmann J, Deuel E, Fanconi S, Haller O (1978) Inborn resistance of mice to myxoviruses: macrophages express phenotype in vitro. J Exp Med 147:531

Lopez C (1979) Immunological nature of genetic resistance of mice of herpes simplex virus type 1 infection. In: De The G, Heule W, Rapp F (eds) Third international symposium on herpes viruses and oncogenesis. WHO Geneva, pp 775–778

Mayer V, Schulman JL, Kilbourne ED (1973) Nonlinkage of neurovirulence exclusively to viral hemagglutinin or neuraminidase in genetic recombinants of A/NWS (NONl) influenza virus. J Virol 11:272

Minato N, Bloom BR, Jones C, Holland J, Reid LM (1979) Mechanism of rejection of virus persistently infected tumor cells by athymic nude mice. J Exp Med 149:1117

Miyoshi K, Gamboa ET, Harter DH, Wolf A, Hsu KC (1971) Influenza virus encephalitis in squirrel monkeys receiving immunosuppressive therapy. J Immunol 106:119

Möller G (ed) (1979) Natural killer cells. Immunol Rev 44

Mouse News Letter (1977) 58:106

Nathenson N, Cole GA (1970) Immunosuppression and experimental infection of the nervous system. Adv Virus Res 16:397

Neighbour PA, Rager-Zisman B, Bloom B (1978) Susceptibility of mice to acute and persistent measles infection. Infect Immun 21:764

Nomura T, Ohsawa N, Tamaoki N, Fujiwara K (eds) (1977) Proceedings of the second international workshop on nude mice. Fischer, Stuttgart New York

Pereira HG, Tumova B, Law VG (1975) Avian influenza A viruses. Bull WHO 32:855

Renton KW, Deloria LB, Mannering GJ (1978) Effects of polyriboinosinic acid-polyribocytidylic acid and a mouse interferon preparation on cytochrome P-450-dependent monooxygenase systems in cultures of primary mouse hepatocytes. Mol Pharmacol 14:672

Repik P, Flamand A, Bishop DHL (1974) Effect of interferon upon primary and secondary transcription of vesicular stomatitis and influenza viruses. J Virol 14:1169

Rusanova NA, Soloview VD (1966) On problem of natural antiviral immunity. The hereditary nature of the resistance mechanism in mice of A2G line to influenza virus. Vopr Virusol 11:398

Sabin AB (1952) Genetic, hormonal and age factors in natural resistance to certain viruses. Ann NY Acad Sci 54:1936

Scher I, Steinberg AD, Berning AK, Paul WE (1975a) X-linked B-lymphocyte immune defect in CBA/N mice. II. Studies of the mechanisms underlying the immune defect. J Exp Med 142:637

Scher I, Ahmed A, Strong DM, Steinberg AD, Paul WE (1975b) X-linked B-lymphocyte immune defect in CBA/HN mice. J Exp Med 141:788

Staats J (1976) Standardized nomenclature for inbred strains of mice: sixth listing. Cancer Res 36:4333

Stewart WE II (1979) The interferon system. Springer, Vienna New York

Stewart WE II, Scott WD, Sulkin SE (1969). Relative sensitivities of viruses to different species of interferon. J Virol 4:147

Stuart-Harris CH (1939) A neurotropic strain of human influenza virus. Lancet I:497

Torrence PF, De Clercq E (1977) Inducers and induction of interferons. Pharmac Ther [B] 2:1

Tovey MG, Begon-Lours J, Gresser I (1974) A method for the scale production of potent interferon preparations. Proc Soc Exp Biol Med 146:809

Trapp BD, Honegger P, Richelson E, Webster FH de (1979) Morphological differentiation of mechanically dissociated fetal rat brain in aggregating cell cultures. Brain Res 160:117

Vallbracht A (1977) Neurovirulenz in einem Influenza-A-Rekombinationssystem. PhD dissertation, University of Tübingen

Virelizier JL, Allison AC (1976) Correlation of persistent mouse hepatitis virus (MHV-3) infection with its effect on mouse macrophage cultures. Arch Virol 50:279

Virelizier JL, Gresser I (1978) Role of interferon in the pathogenesis of viral diseases of mice as demonstrated by the use of anti-interferon serum. J Immunol 120:1616

Virolainen M (1968) Hematopoietic origin of macrophages as studied by chromosome markers in mice. J Exp Med 127:943

Welsh RM (1978) Cytotoxic cells induced during lymphocytic choriomeningitis virus infection of mice. I. Characterization of natural killer cell induction. J Exp Med 148:163

Youngner JS, Thacore HR, Kelly ME (1972) Sensitivity of ribonucleic acid and deoxyribonucleic acid viruses to different species of interferon in cell cultures. J Virol 10:171

Zawatzky R, Hilfenhaus J, Kirchner H (1979) Resistance of nude mice to herpes simplex virus and correlation with in vitro production of interferon. Cell Immunol 47:424

# Role of Macrophages and Interferon in Natural Resistance to Mouse Hepatitis Virus Infection

JEAN-LOUIS VIRELIZIER*

## 1 Introduction

Among the many models of experimental viral infections, the mouse hepatitis virus (MHV) model offers a number of advantages for investigation of the host-virus relationship:

1. MHV infection is a naturally occurring infection in the mouse (*Rowe* et al. 1963); *Broderson* et al. 1976; *Ishida* et al. 1978) and thus is not an artificial model.

2. In the case of mouse hepatitis virus type 3 (MHV-3), the natural resistance is observed to various degrees according to the mouse strain considered (*Virelizier* and *Allison* 1976), with either full susceptibility, full resistance, or semiresistance being present. This provides the opportunity to make correlations with parameters of the immune response in a more precise manner than in other models where only two situations (susceptibility and resistance) are observed.

3. The mouse strains showing variable degrees of susceptibility to MHV-3 (namely, A/J, C3H/He, and C57/BL-6) are well-known inbred strains whose biologic parameters have been thoroughly investigated.

4. MHV infections have been among the first models in which the role of macrophages in host defense have been investigated after the pioneering studies of F. Bang and his colleagues (*Bang* and *Warwick* 1960; *Shif* and *Bang* 1970).

5. MHV-3 induces a very easily recognizable cytopathic effect in mouse macrophage cultures by fusing infected macrophages into multinucleated giant cells (*Malucci* 1965). The appearance of this cytopathic effect closely parallels the intensity of viral replication and thus provides a useful tool for in vitro studies in macrophages from different strains of mice (*Virelizier* and *Allison* 1976).

6. MHV-3 infection is so far the only coronavirus model in which the protective role of interferon in vivo has been demonstrated (*Virelizier* and *Gresser* 1978).

7. Finally, the modification of immune responsiveness during acute or persistent infections has been investigated (*Virelizier* et al. 1976).

These various aspects of MHV-3 infection make this model a useful tool to investigate the mechanisms underlying the natural resistance to this type of virus.

*Groupe d' Immunologic et de Rhumatologie Pédiatriques, INSERM U 132, Hôpital des Enfants-Malades, 149 rue de Sèvres, 75730 Paris Cédex 15, France

## 2 The Pathogenesis of MHV-3 Infection in Various Strains of Mice

MHV-3 is a member of the coronavirus group (*McIntosh* 1974) and was first described in 1956 (*Dick* et al. 1956). Although oral administration is not followed by death, parenteral administration always leads to death in outbred and most inbred mouse strains, regardless of the route of injection (intravenous, intraperitoneal, subcutaneous, or intracerebral). MHV-3 causes a systemic infection, with very high virus titers being found in all organs, including liver, lymphoid organs, brain, kidney, and blood (*Piazza* et al. 1967). After the first cycles of replication within Kuppfer cells, the virus can be visualized by electron microscopy in hepatocytes and in the Disse space between Kuppfer cells and hepatocytes (*Miyai* et al. 1963). During acute infection, tissular lesions are mainly observed in the liver, where a massive necrosis, leading to death within 5 to 10 days, is observed. However, lymphoid organs also show profound modifications, especially the thymus where a rapidly progressing destruction of the cortical, but not the medullary, area is observed as early as 48 h after intraperitoneal virus infection (*Virelizier* et al. 1976). By day 4 after infection, the thymus cortex is completely depopulated. A typical lesion observed in all MHV-3-infected organs is giant cell formation, in which MHV-3 antigens can be found by immunofluorescence. By day 5, necrotic lesions are widely disseminated, especially in the liver (almost entirely destroyed), in lymphoid organs (particularly in the spleen where the marginal zone shows giant cells and necrosis), lymph nodes, and Peyer patches. This lethal, systemic infection is observed in most mouse strains, including Swiss, BALB/C, DBA2, and C57/BL 6 and 10, in which 100% of infected mice die.

In contrast, 100% of mice of the A/J strain survive after parenteral administration of MHV-3, whatever the amount or the route of inoculation (*Virelizier* et al. 1975). Instead of the regular increase observed in susceptible mice until death, MHV-3 replication is efficiently controlled in all A/J organs as early as day 2, and the virus cannot be recovered from any organ by day 7 (*Leprevost* et al. 1975a). The A/J thus proved to be a strain fully resistant to MHV-3.

In the course of our study on the in vivo susceptibility of various mouse strains to MHV-3, we soon discovered that old (10–18 weeks) C3H/He mice resist the acute phase of the disease but develop a chronic illness with progressive neurologic signs (*Virelizier* 1972). A correlation was observed between the clinical evolution and the titer of virus tested during the acute phase of the infection. C3H/He mice show intermediate virus titers in all organs tested by day 4 as compared to susceptible or fully resistant strains (*Leprevost* et al. 1975b). Since C3H/He and A2G mice both develop signs of a chronic neurologic disease, we have investigated the neuropathologic effects of persistent MHV-3 infection in these two strains (*Virelizier* et al. 1975). The majority (75%–95%) of mice from these strains appear normal untill 3–12 weeks after intraperitoneal injection. They then begin to look ill, showing failure to thrive, oily hair and loss of activity. Progressive neurologic signs appear as the mice show incoordination and paresis of one or more limbs. Organ suspensions from chronically sick mice, when injected into susceptible recipients, induce a fulminant hepatitis and a highly virulent virus can be recovered. This indicates that the chronic neurologic disease is associated with the persistence of MHV-3 in its virulent, hepatotropic state. Thus, intraperitoneal inoculation of a nonneurologically adapted strain of MHV-3 into semiresistant mice provides a new model of persistent infection in which persistence is due to a peculiar response of the host but not to an unusual adaptability of the virus. Whereas A2G mice develop mostly a chronic chorio-ependymitis leading to hydromyelia and hydrocephalus, C3H mice suffer mostly from diffuse vasculitis found in kidney, liver, spleen, brain, and spinal cord. As described previously (*Virelizier* et al. 1975), vessel walls show polymorph infiltration, leukocytoclasis, and often fibrinoid necrosis. Both arteries and veins of large and small diameter are affected, but damage is more often seen in veins and venules than in arteries and arterioles. There is also perivascular infiltration of inflammatory cells, sometimes of an almost granulomatous character. Nearby, long ascending and descending tracts are frequently damaged. Both myelin and axis cylinders are destroyed – always in close association with proliferative, perivascular lesions. Viral antigens and immunoglobulins can be found in the walls of damaged vessels. Since no viral antigen is detected in neural cells, it is likely that neurologic damage is the consequence of the systemic vasculitis. Infective virus, found (although at very low titers) in most organs tested by transfer to susceptible recipients, possibly persists within vessel walls. This is clearly different from the situation observed during infection with a neurotropic strain of mouse hepatitis virus (JHM), in which demyelination has been shown to be the direct result of infection of oligodendrocytes (*Weiner* 1973; *Lambert* et al. 1973). Systemic amyloid is found in C3H mice chronically ill for more than 6 months and is a probable consequence of chronic immunologic stimulation associated with virus persistence in the face of an active host response (*Virelizier* et al. 1975).

Thus, various types of host-virus relationship can be observed during MHV-3 infection. As discussed earlier (*Virelizier* 1979b), genetic differences of host resistance are responsible for the different courses observed, ranging from acute disease (either mild or lethal) to persistent viral infection. It is thus important to know which host defense mechanism(s) underlie the genetically determined course of the disease in different inbred strains of mice.

## 3 Virus Restriction in Individual Macrophages as a Possible Obstacle to MHV-3 Spread: The Blood-Organ Barrier

Macrophages can play a vital, although nonspecific role in viral infections. An elegant way to investigate the antiviral role of macrophages in vivo is to inject mice with colloidal silica, which after phagocytosis induces intracellular breakdown of lysosomes leading to death of the macrophages (*Allison* et al. 1966). Using this technique, *Zisman* et al. (1970) have shown that impaired macrophage function is associated with increased spread of herpes simplex virus to the liver parenchyma, with hepatitis and early death resulting. Macrophages may act within virus-induced lesions, since mononuclear cells appear to be selectively recruited into sites of virus multiplication, as shown during Sindbis virus infection (*McFarland* et al. 1972). Macrophages, especially Kuppfer cells lining the sinusoid in the liver, constitute a functionally complete barrier between blood and hepatocytes. *Mims* (1964) has summarized evidence that viruses introduced into the blood stream are taken up by macrophages, where they can be visualized by immunofluorescence. If Kuppfer cells are able to restrict virus replication, the virus will not be able to reach adjacent hepatocytes. Macrophages would thus be ideally suited to form an efficient obstacle to virus spread from blood to organ tissues and could be key cells in natural resistance if their individual resistance to virus replication was genetically determined.

Evidence exists that indicates that natural resistance to various types of MHV is expressed at the level of individual macrophages. *Bang* and *Warwick* (1960) found that adult mice of the Princeton (PRI) strain are susceptible to lethal infection with the Nelson strain of MHV (MHV-2), whereas the C3H strain is resistant. Mating experiments show that susceptibility to infection segregates as a single Mendelian dominant genetic factor. Cultures of hepatic or peritoneal macrophages from mice of susceptible strains support multiplication of MHV-2, whereas macrophages from resistant mice do not. Thus inherited resistance is manifested in vitro in the absence of any specific immune response. This resistance, however, is not a general one to all types of viruses. For example, the PRI mice, which are resistant to arboviruses (*Sabin* 1954), are highly susceptible to MHV-2, and the two resistance factors segregate independently among the offspring of hybrids (*Kantoch* et al. 1963). At an early stage of infection with MHV-2, viral antigen is demonstrable by immunofluorescence in sinusoidal lining cells of the liver and is more prominent in susceptible than in resistant mice (*Taguchi* et al. 1976). In vitro interactions of MHV-2 and macrophages have been investigated by *Shif* and *Bang* (1970). The virus is absorbed equally well to resistant and susceptible cells, but it persists without multiplication in resistant cells, while it disappears into eclipse phase in the susceptible cells and subsequently replicates. Thus a true restriction of virus replication appears to operate. These original observations from *Bang* and his colleagues have been extended in other MHV models. *Allison* (1965) reported that macrophages taken later from neonatally thymectomized animals support the multiplication of the avirulent MHV-1, whereas the virus multiplies to a very limited extent in macrophages from intact adult animals. Using the highly virulent MHV-3, we have shown that there is a precise correlation between the in vitro ability of the virus to grow in macrophages from a given strain of mice and the in vivo course of the disease (*Virelizier* and *Allison* 1976) in the three types of host-virus relationships observed in this model. Thus very little or no virus replication is observed in macrophages from A/J mice in which MHV-3 induces a mild disease with 100% recovery. In cultures of macrophages from susceptible strains (C57/BL, DBA2, etc.), MHV-2 replicates freely, with giant cell formation (see Figure 1), in parallel with the fulminant hepatitis seen in vivo leading to death in 100% of animals. In contrast to this full susceptibility or resistance, macrophage cultures from a strain of mice in which persistent infections occur show intermediate susceptibility, as judged by the intensity of the cytopathic effect, the presence of viral antigens in the cytoplasm, and the levels of viral replication. Thus a genetically controlled "semiresistance" to MHV-3 is manifested in individual macrophages by an intermediate level of viral replication. That macrophages have an antiviral role in vivo during MHV infections has been further suggested by cell transfer experiments. *Stohlman* et al. (1980) have shown that young susceptible mice can be protected from the encephalitis induced by intracranial inoculation with the JHM strain of MHV after transfer of adherent spleen cells from adult resistant animals. Adherent cells were protective even after depletion of T cells before transfer. In contrast, in the MHV-3 model, transfer of resistance from adults to newborn is obtained only when both adherent and nonadherent spleen cells are transferred. Transfer of resistance to MHV-3 is obtained, however, when peritoneal cells are associated with adherent spleen cells (*Levy-Leblond* and *Dupuy* 1977). A third population of bone marrow cells enhances the protective ability of transferred spleen cells (*Tardieu* et al. 1980).

This array of evidence strongly implicates macrophages in natural resistance to MHV and suggests that these cells, being primary targets for the virus, may represent a first line of antiviral defense. However, the precise mechanism(s) through which

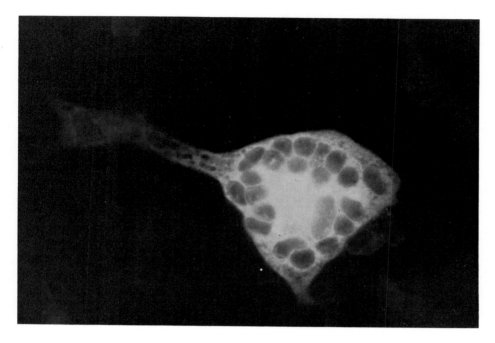

Fig. 1. Multinucleated giant cell observed in culture of adherent peritoneal cells of C57/BL mice infected 48 h previously with MHV-3 (Mill-Hill strain). Note the process of fusion of a single macrophage into a giant cell. Direct immunofluorescence shows viral antigens in cytoplasm, but not in nuclei

macrophages exert this antiviral role in vivo is not yet clear. Restriction of virus replication may not be the only, or even the main, macrophage role during infection. Apart from inactivating virus following endocytosis, mononuclear phagocytes may interfere with virus multiplication and spread through many mechanisms. Firstly, their ability to process and present antigens may facilitate the induction of the specific antiviral cell-mediated response (*Cowing* et al. 1978). Secondly, they may act as nonspecific cytotoxic effector cells able to destroy virus-infected cells, as is suggested in the Semliki Forest virus model (*Rodda* and *White* 1976). Thirdly, macrophages may be major producers of soluble mediators (*Allison* 1978) during viral infections, including interferon (*Glasgow* and *Habel* 1963). *Hirsch* et al. (1970) have shown that peritoneal macrophages transferred from adult CBA mice protect suckling syngeneic mice from intraperitoneal infection with herpes simplex virus. The enhanced resistance provided by stimulated macrophages was associated with more efficient intracellular destruction of virus and with greater production of interferon. Infected macrophages from suckling mice did not produce detectable interferon. Thus, the maturation of antiviral host defense during the first weeks of life correlates with a greater ability of individual macrophages to restrict herpes simplex virus and to produce interferon. Since macrophages are preferential host cells for the first cycle of MHV-3 replication, they could play a decisive antiviral part by producing an early interferon response during infection.

## 4 Protective Role of Early Interferon Production During MHV-3 Infection

Decisive evidence for a protective role of the production of endogenous interferon during viral infections has long been lacking, although administration of exogenous interferon had been shown to confer a marked protection of virus-infected animals under precise experimental conditions (*Finter* 1973; *Baron* 1973). Using an inverse approach, it has more recently been possible to neutralize in vivo the antiviral effects of interferon, a procedure which provides an elegant way to selectively abolish a single component of the host response, namely, endogenous production of interferon during viral infections. *Fauconnier* (1970) has shown that inoculation of sheep anti-mouse interferon serum of low potency was associated with a more rapid onset of disease and an increased mortality in mice infected with Semliki Forest virus. Using a potent antiserum to mouse fibroblast interferon, *Gresser* and his colleagues have provided decisive evidence that interferon plays a major antiviral part in many experimental models. Administration of this antiserum to mice infected with encephalomyocarditis virus resulted in the multiplication of virus to high titers in visceral organs, rapid onset of disease, and early death (*Gresser* et al. 1976a). Similar results were obtained in mice infected with Herpes simplex, Moloney sarcoma, vesicular stomatitis, and Newcastle disease, but not in mice infected with influenza viruses (*Gresser* et al. 1976b).

In the MHV-3 model we have shown that interferon is produced during infection in both resistant (A/J) or susceptible (C57/BL) mice, with peak production of about 1000 units observed 24–48 h after intraperitoneal administration of the virus (*Virelizier* et al. 1976). On the other hand, we have reported that "immune" interferon produced by stimulated leukocytes can inhibit MHV-3 replication in macrophages cultures from susceptible mouse strains (*Virelizier* et al. 1977), an observation which opens up the possibility that immune interferon, as a soluble mediator of specifically sensitized leukocytes, may strengthen the macrophage barrier by inducing an antiviral state in individual cells. *Virelizier* and *Gresser* (1978) have shown that injection of an antiserum to mouse fibroblast interferon before MHV-3 administration accelerates the onset of death in C57/BL mice and induces almost 100% acute mortality in C3H mice, which usually do not die of acute disease (see Fig. 2). Anti-interferon serum administration also causes death in 4- and 6-week-old mice of the resistant strain A/J. These observations demonstrate an important protective role of the endogenous production of "classical" interferon and also show that the efficiency of interferon is variable according to the mouse strain considered. In fully susceptible C57/BL mice, death is observed whether or not interferon has been neutralized, suggesting that interferon production is not sufficient by itself to protect mice and that other factors must be involved which are also critical for recovery. In fully resistant A/J mice, potentiation of infection is clearly noted in young animals (4- to 8-week-old). However, 10- to 22-week-old A/J mice resisted infection whether or not anti-interferon serum was administered. This suggests that endogenous interferon production is essential for protection during the maturation process which transforms susceptible suckling A/J into fully resistant adults during the first 2–3 weeks of life. From then on, another resistance mechanism seems to take over. The possibility exists that A/J macrophages (and/or other cells) have irreversibly acquired the ability to restrict virus replication by the 10$^{th}$ week of life; this maturation process could itself be the consequence of previous production of interferon due to past exposure to bacterial infection in animals which

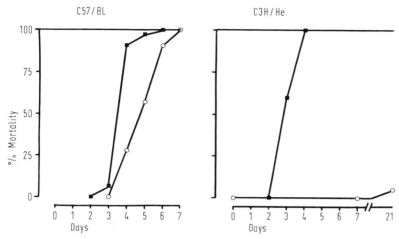

Fig. 2. Mortality observed in mice of the C57/BL (susceptible) or C3H/He (semiresistant) strain infected intraperitoneally with MHV-3 one h after administration of either normal serum (○) or sheep anti-mouse fibroblast interferon (■)

have not been raised under germ-free conditions. In semiresistant C3H mice, interferon production is clearly a critical host defense factor, since injection of anti-interferon serum leads to fulminant hepatitis, whereas control mice develop a chronic neurologic disease associated with virus persistence at very low titers as described above. It should be emphasized that neutralization of circulating interferon during the first 48 h of infection was enough to potentiate the infection, even when interferon was present in the serum at 72 h. This introduces the notion that the fate of MHV-3 infection (chronic disease versus acute hepatitis) is decided very early during infection at a stage when the specific immune response is unlikely to be already operative. Finally, we observed that injection of antiserum into C3H mice chronically infected (2–4 months after virus administration) did not appear to exacerbate the disease. It should be underlined, however, that our antiserum is directed against type I ("classical") virus-induced interferon, so that these results do not preclude a role of type II ("immune") interferon in the chronic disease. Indeed, we have shown that very low titers of interferon circulate in persistently infected C3H mice (*Virelizier* et al. 1976), but the antigenicity of this interferon has not been investigated.

The exact mechanism(s) through which interferon exerts its antiviral activity during MHV-3 or other virus infections is not known. Interferon may induce an antiviral state in every cell of the body or mostly in macrophages. Alternatively, interferon may act through activation of immunologic effectors of immunity (*Virelizier* 1980) such as NK cells (*Gidlund* et al. 1978), cytotoxic macrophages (*Schultz* and *Chirigos* 1979), or cytotoxic T lymphocytes (*Lindahl* et al. 1972).

## 5 Respective Roles of Various Parameters of the Anti-MHV Response

Although it is clear that both interferon and macrophages have a protective role during MHV infection, other factors are possibly involved in host defense mechanisms. The humoral response, however, is unlikely to play a major part, since transfer of serum from immunized A/J mice is not effective in protecting susceptible DBA2 mice against challenge with MHV-3 (*Le Prevost* et al. 1975a). The role of cell-mediated immunity is probably important, in view of the potentiation of infection observed in mice subjected to immunosuppressive drugs. The antiviral role of specific cytotoxic T lymphocytes has not yet been investigated in any MHV model. The possible role of soluble mediators of specifically sensitized T lymphocytes deserves consideration. That viral antigens can induce the secretion of immune interferon has been established with other viruses (*Epstein* et al. 1972; *Valle* et al. 1975) but not yet with MHV antigens.

Various types of immunomanipulation of the host have been used in the hope of obtaining evidence on mechanisms of antiviral defense to MHV in vivo. MHV-2 infection is potentiated by treatment with cortisone (*Gallily* et al. 1964) or cyclophosphamide (*Willenborg* et al. 1973). MHV-3 infection is potentiated by X-ray irradiation or antilymphocyte serum treatment (*Dupuy* et al. 1975). The results of this type of experiment are usually taken as evidence that specific cell-mediated immunity is of major importance in resistance. Other interpretations are possible, however, since immunosuppressive agents do not affect only T lymphocyte functions. For example, we have shown that cortisone, antithymocyte serum, or X-ray irradiation profoundly decreases the production of Sendai virus-induced leukocyte interferon in normal or nude mice (*Virelizier* 1979b), indicating that a non-T-cell-dependent mechanism of host defense is impaired after immunosuppressive treatment. Interestingly, X-ray irradiation breaks resistance to MHV-3 in normal mice, but not in immune A/J mice (*Dupuy* et al. 1975). This is reminiscent of our observation that, whereas nonspecific induction of leukocyte interferon is radiosensitive, the secondary-type secretion of immune interferon by sensitized lymphocytes is radio resistant (*Virelizier* and *Guy-Grand* 1980).

Cell transfer experiments usually involve separation of "macrophages" from "lymphocytes" through cell adherence. Certain cells of the monocyte lineage, however, do not readily adhere to glass or plastic. Promonocytes are nonadherent, nonphagocytic cells, and usually contaminate suspensions of nonadherent lymphocytes. Promonocytes are good candidates for effectors of natural killing (*Lohmann-Mattes* et al. 1979) and leukocyte interferon production (*Virelizier* 1979b). Clearly, cell transfer experiments will benefit from future progress in cell separation and identification.

The immunosuppression observed during viral infections has often been considered as a possible way for a virus to escape the host's immune response. Immune responsiveness is indeed modified during MHV-3 infection (*Virelizier* et al. 1976). However, the role of timing was shown to be critical during acute infection: infecting mice before unrelated antigen (sheep erythrocytes) administration led to immunodepression, whereas simultaneous injection of virus and antigen led to immunostimulation. If this immunologic enhancement also applies to antigens of the infecting virus, the modifications induced by the infection may in fact enhance antiviral responses and thus be beneficial for the host.

# 6 Which Resistance Factor (S) is Genetically Controlled?

As pointed out by *Allison* (1965), inherited differences in susceptibility are sometimes manifested in cell cultures and are thus a property of individual cells. Nevertheless, there may be a synergistic effect with immune mechanisms of the host, so that impairment of the latter greatly increases susceptibility. This is clearly the case in the MHV models, where genetic resistance in individual macrophages is observed in vitro while in vivo resistance can be broken by various immunosuppressive agents, some of which are unlikely to directly affect macrophages. Resistance in the MHV-3 model is under complex, probably polygenic, control (*Levy-Leblond* et al. 1979).

Each effector of the anti-MHV-3 response could be under direct genetic control. The effect of the resistant gene(s) could be exerted on viral restriction by macrophages. Indeed, full susceptibility, full resistance or semiresistance is manifested in vitro in individual macrophages. However, this ability of macrophages to restrict viral replication could itself be under the influence of soluble mediators, the secretion of which would be genetically determined.

Macrophage-mediated cytotoxicity against virus-infected target cells would be an interesting possibility. However, the two mouse strains that resist MHV-3 infection, namely A/J and C3H, show a genetically controlled defect of macrophage tumoricidal capacity (*Boraschi* and *Meltzer* 1979). This hypothesis is thus unlikely if we assume that antiviral and anti-tumor cytotoxic activities of macrophages represent a common phenomenon.

Similarly, natural killer activity is under genetic control in mice and is known to be low in animals of the A/J strain (*Petranyi* et al. 1975).

Genetic differences in interferon production could be involved, since interferon has been shown to have an antiviral role in vivo during MHV-3 infection. However, we could not find significant differences in the titers of circulating interferon in susceptible C57/BL or resistant A/J mice during MHV-3 infection. Furthermore, *De Maeyer* et al. (1975) have reported that A/J mice are among the strains that produce a low circulating interferon response after in vivo induction with Newcastle disease virus, and we have found that A/J leukocytes are low producers of mitogen-induced immune interferon in vitro (unpublished). However, these observations cannot rule out the possibility that macrophages from resistant strains produce an early, but not necessarily intense, interferon response in close contact to neighboring susceptible cells during MHV-3 infection.

Finally, the interesting possibility remains that sensitivity to interferon rather than intensity of interferon production is higher in resistant than in susceptible mice. Such an hypothesis has experimental basis, since cells (including monocytes) from humans with trisomy 21 have an enhanced sensitivity to the antiviral effects of interferon (*Epstein* et al. 1980). A genetically determined difference between strains of mice in sensitivity to interferon has also been suggested by *Haller* et al. (1979). In their model, natural resistance of A2G mice to influenza is manifested in vitro in macrophages and nevertheless can be broken in vivo by administration of anti-interferon serum. In mice resistant to MHV, a high sensitivity to interferon could be shared by all cells of the body or mainly expressed at the level of the macrophage. Endogenous production of interferon, either spontaneous or triggered by immunologic (immune interferon) or infectious (classical interferon) experience, would induce an antiviral state in highly sensitive macrophages from resistant strains, but not in poorly receptive macrophages from susceptible strains. Resistant macrophages, able to resist the first cycle of virus replication, would in turn produce interferon more efficiently. If neighboring hepatocytes also were highly sensitive to interferon, protection would be amplified. Indeed, inborn resistance of mice to MHV 3 has been shown to be expressed in cultured liver parenchymal cells (*Arnheiter* and *Haller*, to be published). Thus sensitivity to interferon produced before and during infection could be a critical factor of recovery. Whatever the exact mechanisms involved, it is probable that intimate interconnection between macrophages and interferon is a major aspect of natural resistance to MHV infection.

# References

Allison AC (1965) Genetic factors in resistance against virus infections. Arch Gesamte Virusforsch 17:280–293

Allison AC (1978) Role of macrophages in the immune response. Immunol Rev 40:3

Allison AC, Harington JS, Birbeck M (1966) An examination of the cytotoxic effects of silica on macrophages. J Exp Med 124:141–153

Arnheiter H, Haller O (to be published) Inborn resistance of mice to mouse hepatitis virus type 3 (MHV-3): liver parenchymal cell express phenotype in culture. In: Biochemistry and biology of coronaviruses

Bang FB, Warwick A (1960) Mouse macrophages as host cells for the mouse hepatitis virus and the genetic basis of their susceptibility. Proc Natl Acad Sci USA 46:1065–1075

Baron S (1973) The defensive and biological roles of the interferon system. Front Biol 2:267–280

Boraschi D, Meltzer MS (1979) Defective tumoricidal capacity of macrophages from A/J mice. II: Comparison of the macrophage cytotoxic defect of A/J mice with of lipid A-unresponsive C3H/HeJ mice. J Immunol 122:1592–1597

Broderson JR, Murphy FA, Hierholzer JC (1976) Lethal enteritis in infant mice caused by mouse hepatitis virus. Lab Anim Sci 26:824–827

Cowing C, Pincus SH, Sachs DH, Dickler HB (1978) A subpopulation of adherent accessory cells bearing both I-A and I-E or C subregion antigens is required for antigen specific murine T lymphocyte proliferation. J Immunol 121:1680–1685

De Maeyer E, Jullien P, De Maeyer-Guignard J, Demant P (1975) Effect of mouse genotype on interferon production. II: Distribution of If-1 alleles among inbred strains and transfer of phenotype by grafting bone marrow cells. Immunogenetics 2:151–160

Dick GWA, Niven JSF, Gledhill AW (1956) A virus related to that causing hepatitis in mice. Br J Exp Pathol 37:90–95

Dupuy JM, Levy-Leblond E, Le Prevost C (1975) Immunopathology of mouse hepatitis virus type 3 infection. II. Effect of immunosuppression in resistant mice. J Immunol 114:226–230

Epstein LB, Stevens DA, Merigan TC (1972) Selective increase in lymphocyte interferon response to vaccinia antigen after revaccination. J Clin Invest 50:744–753

Epstein LB, Lee SHS, Epstein CJ (1980) Enhanced sensitivity of trisomy 21 monocytes to the maturation-inhibiting effect of interferon. Cell Immunol 50:191–194

Fauconnier B (1970) Augmentation de la pathogénicité virale par l'emploi de sérum anti-interféron in vivo. CR Acad Sci [D] (Paris) 271:1466–1470

Finter NB (1973) Interferons and inducers in vivo. I. Antiviral effects in experimental animals. Front Biol 2:135–150

Gallily R, Warwick A, Bang FB (1964) Effect of cortisone on genetic resistance to mouse hepatitis virus in vivo and in vitro. Proc Natl Acad Sci USA 51:1158–1164

Gidlund M, Orn A, Wigzell H, Senik A, Gresser I (1978) Enhanced NK cell activity in mice injected with interferon and interferon inducers. Nature 273:759–761

Glasgow LA, Habel K (1963) Interferon production by mouse leucocytes in vitro and in vivo. J Exp Med 117:149–155

Gresser I, Tovey MG, Bandu MT, Maury C, Brouty-Boye D (1976a) Role of interferon in the pathogenesis of virus diseases in mice as demonstrated by the use of anti-interferon serum. I. Rapid evolution of encephalomyocarditis virus infection. J Exp Med 144:1305–1315

Gresser I, Tovey MG, Maury C, Bandu MT (1976b) Role of interferon in the pathogenesis of virus diseases in mice as demonstrated by the use of anti-interferon serum. II. Studies with Herpes simplex, Moloney sarcoma, Vesicular stomatitis, Newcastle disease and influenza viruses. J Exp Med 114:1316–1323

Haller O, Arnheiter H, Gresser I, Lindenmann J (1979) Genetically determined, interferon-dependent resistance to influenza virus in mice. J Exp Med 149:601–612

Hirsch MS, Zisman B, Allison AC (1970) Macrophages and age dependent resistance to herpes simplex virus in mice. J Immunol 104:1160–1165

Ishida T, Taguchi F, Lee Y, Yamada A, Tamura T, Fujiwara K (1978) Isolation of mouse hepatitis virus from infant mice with fatal diarrhea. Lab Anim Sci 28:269–276

Kantoch M, Warwick A, Bang FB (1963) Cellular nature of genetic susceptibility to a virus. J Exp Med 117:781–797

Lampert PW, Sims JK, Kniazeff AJ (1973) Mechanism of demyelination in JHM virus encephalomyelitis. Electron microscopic studies. Acta Neuropathol (Berl) 24:76–85

Le Prevost C, Levy-Leblond E, Virelizier JL, Dupuy JM (1975a) Immunopathology of mouse hepatitis virus type 3 infection. I. Role of humoral and cellmediated immunity in resistance mechanisms. J Immunol 114:221–225

Le Prevost C, Virelizier JL, Dupuy JM (1975b) Immunopathology of mouse hepatitis virus type 3 infection. III. Clinical and virologic observation of a persistent viral infection. J Immunol 115:640–645

Levy-Leblond E, Dupuy JM (1977) Neonatal susceptibility to MHV-3 infection in mice. I. Transfer off resistance. J Immunol 118:1219–1222

Levy-Leblond E, Oth D, Dupuy JM (1979) Genetic study of mouse sensitivity to MHV-3 infection: influence of the H2 complex. J Immunol 122:1359–1362

Lindahl P, Leary P, Gresser I (1972) Enhancement by interferon of the specific cytotoxicity of sensitized lymphocytes. Proc Natl Acad Sci USA 69:721–725

Lohmann-Mattes ML, Domizig W, Roder J (1979) Promonocytes have the functional characteristics of natural killer cells. J Immunol 123:1883–1887

McFarland HF, Griffin DE, Johnson RT (1972) Specificity of the inflammatory response in viral encephalitis. I. Adoptive immunization of immunosuppressed mice with Sindbis virus. J Exp Med 136:216–220

McIntosh K (1974) Coronaviruses: a comparative review. Curr Top Microbiol Immunol 63:85–129

Malucci L (1965) Observations on the growth of mouse hepatitis virus (MHV-3) in mouse macrophages. Virology 25:30–37

Mims CA (1964) Aspects of the pathogenesis of virus disease. Bacteriol Rev 28:30–71

Miyai K, Slusser RJ, Ruebner BH (1963) Viral hepatitis in mice: an electron microscopic study. Exp Mol Pathol 2:464–480

Petranyi GG, Kiessling R, Klein G (1975) Genetic control of natural killer lymphocytes in the mouse. Immunogenetics 2:53–61

Piazza M, Pane G, De Ritis F (1977) The fate of MHV-3 after intravenous injection into susceptible mice. Arch Gesamte Virusforsch 22:472–474

Roda SJ, White DO (1976) Cytotoxic macrophages: a rapid nonspecific response to viral infection. J Immunol 117:2067–2072

Rowe WP, Hartley JW, Capps WI (1963) Mouse hepatitis virus infection as a highly contagious, prevalent, enteric infection in mice. Proc Soc Exp Biol Med 112:161–165

Sabin AB (1954) Genetic factors affecting susceptibility and resistance to virus disease of the nervous system. Ass Res New Ment Dis Proc 33:57–65

Schultz RM, Chirigos MA (1979) Selective neutralization by anti-interferon globulin of macrophage activation by L-cell interferon, Brucella abortus ether extract, Salmonella typhimurium lipopolysaccharide and polyanions. Cell Immunol 48:52–58

Shif I, Bang FB (1970) In vitro interaction of mouse hepatitis virus and macrophages from genetically resistant mice. I. Adsorption of virus and growth curve. J Exp Med 131:843–850

Stohlman SA, Frelinger JA, Weiner LP (1980) Resistance to fatal central nervous system disease by mouse hepatitis virus, strain JHM. II. Adherent cell-mediated protection. J Immunol 124:1733–1739

Taguchi F, Hirano N, Kiuchi Y, Fujiwara K (1976) Difference in response to mouse hepatitis virus among susceptible mouse strains. Japan J Microbiol 20:293–302

Tardieu M, Hery C, Dupuy JM (1980) Neonatal susceptibility to MHV-3 infection in mice. II. Role of natural effector marrow cells in transfer of resistance. J Immunol 124:418–423

Valle MJ, Bobrove AM, Strober S, Merigan TC (1975) Immune specific production of interferon by human T cells in combined macrophage-lymphocyte cultures in response to herpes simplex antigen. J Immunol 114:435–441

Virelizier JL (1972) Etude virologique et immunologique d'une virose persistante chez la souris infectée par le virus de l'hépatite murine (MHV-3). MD dissertation, University of Paris-Sud

Virelizier JL (1979a) Pathogenesis of mouse hepatitis virus (MHV-3) infection in various inbred strains of mice. In: Bachmann PA (ed) Mechanisms of viral pathogenesis and virulence. WHO, München, p 251

Virelizier JL (1979b) Effects of immunosuppressive agents on leucocyte interferon production in normal or thymus-deprived mice. Transplantation 27:353–355

Virelizier JL (1980) Immunological aspects of interferon secretion. In: Collier LH, Oxford J (eds) Developments in antiviral chemotherapy. Academic Press, London New York, p 201

Virelizier JL, Allison AC (1976) Correlation of persistent mouse hepatitis (MHV-3) infection with its effect on mouse macrophage cultures. Arch Virol 50:279–285

Virelizier JL, Gresser I (1978) Role of interferon in the pathogenesis of viral diseases of mice as demonstrated by the use of anti-interferon serum. V. Protective role in mouse hepatitis virus type 3 infection of susceptible and resistant strains of mice. J Immunol 120:1616–1619

Virelizier JL, Guy-Grand D (1980) Immune interferon secretion as an expression of immunological memory to transplantation antigens: in vivo generation of long-lived, recirculating memory cells. Eur J Immunol 10:375–379

Virelizier JL, Dayan AD, Allison AC (1975) Neuropathological effects of persistent infection of mice by mouse hepatitis virus. Infect 12:1127–1140

Virelizier JL, Virelizier AM, Allison AC (1976) The role of circulating interferon in the modifications of immune responsiveness by mouse hepatitis virus (MHV-3). J Immunol 117:748–753

Weiner LP (1973) Pathogenesis of demyelination induced by a mouse hepatitis virus (JHM virus). Arch Neurol 28:298–303

Willenborg DO, Shan KV, Bang FB (1973) Effect of cyclophosphamide on the genetic resistance of C3H mice to mouse hepatitis virus. Proc Soc Exp Biol Med 142:762–766

Zisman B, Hirsch MS, Allison AC (1970) Selective effects of anti-macrophage serum, silica and anti-lymphocyte serum on pathogenesis of herpes virus infection of young adult mice. J Immunol 104:1155–1159

# Genetic Resistance to Friend Virus-Induced Erythroleukemia and Immunosuppression

Vinay Kumar and Michael Bennett*

## 1 Introduction

The Friend virus (FV) is a complex of a replication-defective spleen focus forming virus (SFFV) and its helper lymphatic leukemia virus (LLV) (*Steeves* et al. 1971; *Troxler* et al. 1977). Infection of susceptible adult mice with FV leads to a rapidly developing erythroleukemia accompanied by extensive viral replication in the spleen and profound suppression of humoral and cellular immunity (*Bennett* and *Steeves* 1970; *Mortensen* et al. 1974). Within 7–9 days after infection with small doses of FV, the spleen becomes enlarged due mainly to focal proliferation of neoplastic erythroid cells. This results in the characteristic appearance of raised yellowish foci when such spleens are fixed in Bouin's solution (*Axelrad* and *Steeves* 1964). As the disease progresses, both liver and spleen enlarge, but thymus and lymph nodes remain relatively unaffected. One variant of FV, isolated initially by Mirand (*Mirand* et al. 1968), leads to a progressive increase in hematocrit (polycythemia), and eventually most mice die, often with splenic rupture, in 30–60 days. Several H-2-linked and nonlinked genes which regulate the effects of FV have been described. The *Fv-1* locus controls host resistance to the helper virus. *Fv-1*-mediated re-

*Department of Pathology, Boston University School of Medicine, Boston, Mass. 02118, USA

sistance is not unique to Friend LLV but rather a general phenomenon seen with respect to a variety of murine leukemia virus (MuLV) isolates (*Pincus* et al. 1971). Two alleles designated as $Fv$-$1^n$ and $Fv$-$1^b$ have been described and these define the N or B tropism of MuLV. The $Fv$-$1$ gene regulates viral replication, and it is possible to overcome $Fv$-$1$ resistance by utilizing laboratory-derived NB-tropic viruses. We chose to utilize an NB-tropic stock of FV complex, since we were primarily interested in the study of host resistance to SFFV. The $Fv$-$2$ locus controls resistance to the spleen focus forming virus (*Lilly* 1970). Adult homozygous resistant mice ($Fv$-$2^{r/r}$) are completely resistant to spleen focus formation and erythroleukemia induction. Such mice belong mainly to the C57BL family, i.e., C57BL/10, C57BL/6, B6, and B10 $H$-$2$ congenics and C58 mice. Such mice are also relatively resistant to the immunosuppressive effects of FV. Both viral replication and immunosuppression in $Fv$-$2^{r/r}$ mice are transient and significantly lesser in magnitude as compared with $Fv$-$2^{s/s}$ mice (*Ceglowski* and *Friedman* 1969). The $Fv$-$2$ gene is unlinked to $H$-$2$ and has been mapped on chromosome 9. $Fv$-$2$ susceptibility is dominant over resistance (unlike the $Fv$-$1$ gene). Although $Fv$-$2^{r/r}$ mice are resistant to the immunosuppressive effects of FV, our studies have indicated that genetic susceptibility to the immunosuppressive effect of FV is mediated by a gene distinct from $Fv$-$2$, called $Fv$-$3$. The $Fv$-$3$ gene is discussed later in this review. While $Fv$-$2$ regulates the susceptibility of induction to Friend erythroleukemia, a series of $H$-$2$-linked genes regulates the recovery from leukemia in $Fv$-$2^{s/s}$ or $Fv$-$2^{r/s}$ mice. Elegant studies by Chesebro and colleagues have defined at least three $Rfv$ (recovery from Friend virus) genes, two of which are linked to $H$-$2$ (*Chesebro* et al. 1974; *Chesebro* and *Wehrly* 1978; *Chesebro* and *Wehrly* 1979). These will not be discussed in this review. Instead we will focus our discussion on the mechanism of action of the $Fv$-$2$ and $Fv$-$3$ genes.

## 2 Possible Mechanism of $Fv$-$2^{r/r}$-Mediated Resistance

Resistance to leukemogenesis by FV could be due either to resistance of the "target cells" to the transforming effects of FV, or alternatively the resistance could be immunologically mediated. The latter implies that the erythropoietic stem cells of $Fv$-$2^{r/r}$ mice may be susceptible to transformation by FV, but the transformed, malignant cells would be attacked and eliminated by the immune system. Several lines of evidence favor the concept of target cell resistance. Suppression of the T cell system either by thymectomy or by antilymphocyte serum fails to render genetically resistant mice susceptible to leukemia or to immunosuppression (*Stutman* and *Dupuy* 1972). Suppression of antibody synthesis by administration of cortisol also fails to confer susceptibility on resistant mice (*Bennett* and *Steeves* 1970). Indeed, suppression of B cells by prolonged administration of anti-IgM antibodies renders $Fv$-$2^{s/s}$ mice resistant to leukemia induction (*Manning* et al. 1974). Therefore B cells may be essential for FV leukemogenesis. Administration of silica, a macrophage poison, also fails to overcome genetic resistance (*Kumar* and *Bennett*, unpublished work). Genetic resistance ($Fv$-$2^{r/r}$) or susceptibility ($Fv$-$2^{s/s}$) could be transferred by $H$-$2$-compatible bone marrow cell transplants (*Odaka* and *Matsukura* 1969). This indicates that resistance is a property intrinsic to the hemopoietic cells and supports the concept that $Fv$-$2$ affects target cells directly (*Axelrad* and *Van Der Gaag* 1968). However, these earlier studies had not considered the possible host defense role of those effector cells which are responsible for rejection of bone marrow allografts (*Cudkowicz* and *Bennett* 1971a, b). The effector cells responsible for genetic resistance against hemopoietic cell allografts differ from T and B cells in several respects. These cells do not require thymic influence for maturation; indeed, athymic nude mice are better than littermate controls in their ability to reject incompatible bone marrow grafts. There is no evidence for the involvement of humoral antibodies in the rejection of hemopoietic transplants, and conventional means of B cell suppression do not affect marrow allograft reactivity (*Hochman* and *Cudkowicz* 1977). Rejection of bone marrow allografts can occur after whole-body lethal irradiation in unprimed mice, suggesting that the effector cells in vivo are naturally "programmed." If any further inductive steps are required, they do not require cell proliferation. The target antigens involved in the rejection of bone marrow allografts are also distinct from the conventional codominantly inherited transplantation antigens. These have been called *hemopoietic* or *hybrid histocompatibility* (*Hh*) antigens and are expressed primarily on normal hemopoietic stem cells (*Cudkowicz* and *Bennett* 1971a, b; *Bennett* 1972; *Lotzova* 1977). Immune-response-like genes, not linked to *H-2*, regulate the anti-*Hh* response of various inbred mouse strains (*Cudkowicz* 1971). Several agents are known to suppress these effector cells. These include macrophage stimulants such as heat-killed *Corynebacterium parvum* organisms (*Cudkowicz* and *Bennett* 1971a, b), macrophage poisons such as silica or carrageenans (*Lotzova* and *Cudkowicz* 1974; *Cudkowicz* and *Yung* 1977), cyclophosphamide (*Cudkowicz* and *Bennett* 1971), $^{89}$Sr (*Bennett* 1973), and estradiol (*Seaman* et al. 1979). $^{89}$Sr is of particular interest, since this agent is rather selective in its action. Administration of $^{89}$Sr to mice profoundly suppresses their ability to reject incompatible bone marrow grafts, without elimination of the major elements of the immune system (B cells, T cells, macrophages).

## 2.1 Effect of $^{89}$Sr Administration on Genetic Resistance to Friend Virus

Several lines of evidence suggest a similarity between effector cells responsible for marrow allograft reactivity and those responsible for genetic resistance to SFFV (*Bennett* and *Eckner* 1973): 1. There is a considerable, but not absolute, overlap between strains of mice that could be classed as "good responders" to most bone marrow allografts and as resistant to the leukemogenic and immunosuppressive effects of FV. 2. Friend erythroleukemic cells of DBA/2 origin show enhanced expression of certain *Hh* antigens (*Rossi* et al. 1973). 3. Ability to reject bone marrow allografts develops rather late, i.e., after 3 weeks, and even $Fv-2^{r/r}$ mice are sensitive to the effects of FV before 3 weeks of age. In view of these similarities, the effect of $^{89}$Sr administration on the genetic resistance to the effects of FV was tested (Table 1). Adult C57BL/6 ($Fv-2^{r/r}$) mice were injected twice with 100 µCi $^{89}$Sr 4 weeks apart. Six weeks after the second injection, mice were infected with NB-tropic FV and transfused with red blood cells (RBC) to inhibit physiologic erythropoiesis. Nine days after infection the $^{89}$Sr-treated mice developed massive splenomegaly, although no discrete foci of neoplastic cells could be seen on the surface. The histology showed diffuse replacement of the spleen by erythroblasts even after transfusion. In addition, $^{89}$Sr-treated B6 mice, unlike control B6 mice and like $Fv-2^{s/s}$ mice, supported extensive viral replication in the spleen and blood. Their ability to mount an anti-sheep red blood cell (SRBC) antibody response was also markedly suppressed. Thus by the above criteria, the $Fv-2^{r/r}$ B6 mice were converted phenotypically into genetically susceptible mice (*Kumar* et al. 1974). These mice have not been followed

Table 1. Effect of $^{89}$Sr on genetic resistance of C57BL/6 mice to FV-induced erythroleukemia

| Treatment with $^{89}$Sr[a] | Infection with FV[a] | Erythroid cells in spleen[a] | Virus recovery in | |
|---|---|---|---|---|
| | | | Spleen | Plasma |
| | | % | FFU/Spleen | FFU/ml |
| Yes | Yes | 95 | $> 10^5$ | $> 10^5$ |
| Yes | No | 3 | 0 | 0 |
| No | Yes | 1.5 | 0 | 0 |
| No | No | 0.3 | NT | NT |

[a] C57BL/6 adult mice with or without prior treatment with $^{89}$Sr were infected with 100 FFU of NB-tropic FV. On days 5 and 6 after infection (or not) with FV, mice were infused with 1 ml whole mouse blood intravenously to suppress physiologic erythropoiesis. Nine days after infection mice were killed. Plasma and spleens were removed at this time for various assays. Details in *Kumar* et al. 1974

for long periods of time, and hence it is not possible to state whether $^{89}$Sr treatment had also overcome the effect of *Rfv* resistance genes. Furmanski and colleagues inoculated control and $^{89}$Sr-treated Swiss mice (*Fv-2^{s/s}*) with an FV variant normally associated with a high incidence of recovery. The incidence of recovery was markedly reduced in the $^{89}$Sr-treated mice (*Furmanski* et al. 1979).

## 2.2 Transformation of *Fv-2^{r/r}* Erythroid Progenitor Cells

The data with $^{89}$Sr-treated B6 mice suggested that the effector system responsible for marrow allograft reactivity may also be involved in surveillance against FV. However, since $^{89}$Sr treatment causes considerable changes in hemopoiesis (see Sect. 3), this data cannot rule out the target cell hypothesis completely. To ask the question whether erythropoietic stem cells from *Fv-2^{r/r}* mice can be transformed by FV in the absence of $^{89}$Sr treatment, DBA/2 (*Fv-2^{s/s}*, *H-2^d*) mice were infected with a large dose of FV. Four days later they were lethally irradiated. Bone marrow cells from B10.D2 (*Fv-2^{r/r}*, *H-2^d*) mice were transplanted into such mice to allow for possible transformation of *Fv-2^{r/r}* cells in the leukemic "susceptible microenvironment". Five to 30 days later spleens of DBA/2 recipients were retransplanted into unirradiated adult B10.D2 secondary recipients to assay for tumor-colony-forming units (TCFU) of B10.D2 origin. Using this "two-step" system, it was possible to detect transformed cells of B10.D2 origin in the spleens of irradiated infected DBA/2 mice, suggesting that *Fv-2^{r/r}* cells can be transformed under appropriate conditions (Table 2; *Kumar* et al. 1974). It should be noted that the TCFU assay employed by us differs from the one in which it was found that tumor colonies seen in the recipient mice were of host rather than donor origin (*Steeves* et al. 1978).

## 3 Effect of $^{89}$Sr Administration on Immune Functions

Treatment with $^{89}$Sr, but none of the other immunosuppressive regimens tested, can override the genetic resistance to FV leukemia. It is therefore important to consider the

Table 2. Transformation of B10.D2 bone marrow cells (BMC) in spleens of leukemic irradiated DBA/2 Mice (*Kumar* et al. 1974)[a]

| Experiment | No. of B10.D2 BMC transplanted | Virus infection of DBA/2 pri- mary recipient | No. of days be- tween B10.D2 BMC transplan- tation and assay for TCFU | No. of TCFU recovered |
|---|---|---|---|---|
| 1 | $10^7$ | + | 7 | > 100 |
|   | $10^7$ | − | 7 | 0 |
|   | No cells | + | 5 | 0 |
| 2 | $10^6$ | + | 5 | 35.0 |
|   | $10^6$ | + | 15 | 27.0 |
|   | $10^6$ | + | 30 | 0 |

[a] DBA/2 primary recipient mice were infected with FV. Four days later they were irradiated (800 R) and transplanted with B10.D2 BMC. At various later intervals the tumor colony form- ing unit (TCFU) content of the DBA/2 spleens was assayed as described

effects of [89]Sr administration on the lymphohematopoietic tissues of mice. [89]Sr is an iso- tope which is selectively incorporated in the bones and irradiates the bone marrow cavity with β-rays (*Fried* et al. 1966). Owing to its relatively long half-life (59 days), even a single administration of [89]Sr leads to chronic irradiation of the marrow cavity. In [89]Sr-treated mice bone marrow is rendered hypoplastic and the spleen takes over stem cell functions (*Gurney* et al. 1972). The spleens are often moderately enlarged, and histologically the red pulp shows very active myelopoiesis. The thymus and lymph nodes are normal histologi- cally, except for the presence of occasional foci of granulopoiesis and increased mast cell numbers (*Bennett* et al. 1976).

## 3.1 T- and B-Cell Functions in [89]Sr-Treated Mice

In the *resting* state a variety of T-cell functions measured in [89]Sr-treated mice are either normal or modestly suppressed. Alloreactive T-cell function has been measured by the ability of [89]Sr-treated mice to reject skin grafts (*Gurney* et al. 1972), the ability of lymph node cells to mediate graft-versus-host reactions in irradiated recipients (*Bennett* 1973), and the ability of spleen cells to generate cytotoxic alloreactive T cells (CTL) and mixed lymphocyte cultures. All these functions are relatively normal in [89]Sr-treated mice, ex- cept for the occasional modest reduction in the generation of CTL (*Kumar* and *Bennett,* unpublished work). T cells obtained from [89]Sr-treated mice are fully competent to provide helper function to B cells in the anti-SRBC plaque-forming cell (PFC) response when tested  in a cell transfer system (*Bennett* 1973). Recent experiments suggest that spleen cells from [89]Sr-treated mice are deficient in their ability to generate macrophage- activating factors (MAF) in response to stimulation with concanavalin A (ConA) (*Masu- da* and *Bennett,* to be published). Since the production of MAF is usually ascribed to a splenic T cell, these results indicate a quantitative or a qualitative defect in certain splenic T cells. CTL responses to syngeneic tumor cells and to parental-strain spleen cells are also defective (*Fitzgerald* and *Bennett,* submitted; *Luevano* et al., to be published).

[89]Sr-treated mice immunized with SRBC generate normal numbers of anti-SRBC plaque-forming cells in vivo. In cell transfer experiments precursor B cells in the [89]Sr-treated mice generate normal numbers of antigen-reactive B cells. The mitogenic response to lipopolysaccharide and dextran sulfate is normal, as is the frequency of 19S EAC rosette-forming cells (*Bennett* et al. 1976).

## 3.2 Macrophage Functions

Accessory cell function as measured by ability to support humoral antibody synthesis is normal in [89]Sr-treated mice (*Bennett* et al. 1976). Peritoneal macrophages from [89]Sr-treated display normal phagocytic and bactericidal activity against *Listeria monocytogenes* when activated by lymphokines and express Ia antigens and Fc and C3b receptors normally (*Masuda* and *Bennett*, unpublished observations). Antibody-dependent cellular cytotoxicity (ADCC) against nucleated red blood cells, presumably mediated by macrophages, is unaffected and the frequency of splenic 7S EA rosette-forming cells is also normal (*Bennett* et al. 1976).

## 3.3 Suppressor Cells in [89]Sr-Treated Mice

Although a variety of T cell, B cell, and macrophage numbers are normal in *resting* [89]Sr-treated mice, it is relatively easy to *activate* suppressor cells. As will be discussed in Sect. 6.4, Friend virus infection of [89]Sr-treated mice can activate T cells capable of suppressing mitogen responses and antibody synthesis. Overnight culture of spleen cells from [89]Sr-treated mice in medium containing fetal calf serum can activate/induce suppressor cells capable of inhibiting in vitro as well as in vivo antibody synthesis (*Merluzzi* et al. 1978). The nature of these cells is not known at the present time. The basis of increased suppressor cell potential in [89]Sr-treated mice is not known. It could result either from a change in the patterns of hemopoiesis resulting from ablation of the bone marrow or alternatively from the loss of certain regulatory cells following [89]Sr treatment.

## 3.4 Natural Killer Cells in [89]Sr-Treated Mice

Natural killer (NK) cells, which have been discussed in detail elsewhere in this volume (see p 107–123), have been considered potentially important in immune surveillance against tumors. These cells, which do not appear to be classical T cells, B cells, or macrophages, share several characteristics with the effector cells responsible for marrow allograft reactivity (*Kiessling* et al. 1977). As mentioned previously, marrow allograft reactivity is abrogated following treatment of mice with [89]Sr. A similar profound suppression of NK cell reactivity against YAC-1 lymphoma cells occurs in [89]Sr-treated mice (*Haller* and *Wigzell* 1977; *Kumar* et al. 1979a, b). A limited survey of NK cell reactivity against a variety of tumor cell targets indicates that [89]Sr treatment does not suppress NK function against all targets. NK activity against YAC-1 (*H-2$^a$* T lymphoma), RL♂-1 (*H-2$^d$* T lymphoma), and MPC-11 (*H-2$^d$* myeloma) is reduced following [89]Sr treatment, whereas reactivity against EL-4 (*H-2$^b$* T lymphoma), FLD-3 (*H-2$^d$* erythroleukemia), WEHI-164 (*H-2$^d$*

sarcoma), and Meth A sarcoma ($H\text{-}2^d$ fibrosarcoma) is not affected to any great extent. In addition, serologic and ontogenetic data (*Burton* et al., to be published; *Bennett* et al., to be published) point to heterogeneity within the NK cells population. Evidence has been presented to support the notion that NK and ADCC activity against tumor cells is mediated by similar cells (*Ojo* and *Wigzell* 1978; *Santoni* et al. 1979). Results with [89]Sr-treated mice support such a concept, since ADCC against EL-4 tumor cells is markedly deficient in spleen cells from [89]Sr-treated mice (*Bennett* et al., to be published).

The mechanism of low NK activity in [89]Sr-treated mice is poorly understood. It has been suggested that bone marrow may be a unique and exclusive source of NK cell precursors (*Haller* and *Wigzell* 1977; *Haller* et al. 1977). Other investigators have suggested that NK cell function is exquisitely susceptible to negative regulation by suppressor cells and that [89]Sr-treated mice possess cells capable of suppressing NK cells at the effector level (*Cudkowicz* and *Hochman* 1979). Our own experiments, details of which are presented elsewhere (*Kumar* et al. 1979a; *Luevano* et al., to be published; *Levy* et al. 1980), indicate the following:

1. [89]Sr-treated mice do not seem to possess suppressor cells for NK (YAC-1) at the effector level either in the resting state or following challenge with tumor cells. 2. In cell transfer experiments, spleen cells from [89]Sr-treated mice fail to suppress the generation of NK cells from their precursors in normal bone marrow or in normal spleen. 3. Normal bone marrow cell infusions fail to restore NK (YAC-1) activity of [89]Sr-treated mice. 4. Spleen cells of [89]Sr-treated mice contain a normal frequency of NK cell precursors. 5. Spleens of [89]Sr-treated mice possess a normal frequency of cells capable of binding to YAC-1 target cells. 6. Spleen cells from mice injected with [89]Sr (two injections of 100 µCi) fail to be stimulated to achieve significant levels of cytotoxicity against YAC-1 by in vivo administration of preparations containing type I or type II interferon and also fail to be stimulated by type I interferon in vitro. The refractoriness to interferon persists even if [89]Sr-treated mice have been reconstituted earlier with normal bone marrow cells. 7. Implantation of normal syngeneic bone fragments into the spleens of [89]Sr-treated mice significantly restores their NK cell activity.

On the basis of these observations we favor the view that NK (YAC-1) cells are dependent upon the normal bone marrow microenvironment for differentiation into a fully lytic and interferon-responsive state. Since bone marrow may be considered a central lymphoid organ for NK (YAC-1) cell differentiation, these cells may be classified as marrow-dependent (M) cells. Cells reactive against hemopoietic cell grafts in vivo may also be M cells.

# 4 M Cells and Genetic Resistance to Leukemia

Erythroid progenitor cells of $Fv\text{-}2^{r/r}$ mice do not seem to be intrinsically resistant to transformation by FV, and abrogation of M-cell function by [89]Sr renders $Fv\text{-}2^{r/r}$ mice susceptible to leukemogenesis. It is therefore plausible that M cells may mediate the effects of $Fv\text{-}2$ in vivo. The susceptibility of infant $Fv\text{-}2^{r/r}$ mice (< 3 weeks old) to leukemia induction is also consistent with such a hypothesis, since infant mice lack M-cell function (both when measured by marrow allograft reactivity in vivo and NK (YAC-1) function in vitro). Stem cells transformed by FV show enhanced expression of certain $Hh$ antigens (*Rossi* et al. 1973), and $Hh$ antigens are known to be the target antigens for M cells in vivo (*Cudkowicz* and *Bennett* 1971a, b). Two possibilities exist for the mechanism of $Fv\text{-}2$ gene function in such a model system: (1) The $Fv\text{-}2^{r/r}$ allele could be an *immune-response*-like gene conferring "a good responder" status on the M cells reactive against the altered/enhanced expression of *Hh* antigens present on the surface of cells transformed by FV; or (2) *Fv-2* could code for certain *Hh*-like antigens expressed only after transformation by FV or could regulate the expression of *Hh* antigens which are normally present on stem cells. In either case $Fv$-$2^{r/r}$ allele would favor the expression of *Hh* antigens in a form immunogenic for the M cells. If this hypothesis is correct, it is conceivable that there exists an in vitro (NK-like) counterpart of the M cells reactive against FV-transformed cells. Although NK (YAC-1) cells do appear to be M cells, it is *unlikely* that the very same cells which lyse YAC-1 in vitro are also reactive against FV erythroleukemia cells in vivo. The strongest argument in favor of this view is that NK reactivity against YAC-1 cells is under polygenic control and *Fv-2* does not appear to be in any way related to the genetic regulation of NK (YAC-1) function. For example, $Fv$-$2^{s/s}$ CBA/J mice have high NK activity against YAC-1, whereas A/J mice which are also $Fv$-$2^{s/s}$ have low NK (YAC-1) activity. If NK cells are monoclonal (a point which is still not settled), one would not even expect NK (YAC-1) to reflect the function of anti-FV cells in vivo. This does not preclude the possibility that NK (YAC-1) cells and cells responsible for genetic resistance against FV are both M cells, albeit distinct subsets. One has only to look at T cells for such a precedence. An NK assay utilizing FLD-3 (Friend erythroleukemia cells of BALB/c origin) has been developed. The killing of FLD-3 cells is not regulated by the *Fv-2* gene (*Lust* et al. 1980). Indeed, significant killing of FLD-3 is seen by spleen cells of syngeneic BALB/c mice, suggesting the presence of some resistance mechanism even in syngeneic hosts. FLD-3 cells maintained in vitro for a long time may have acquired target determinants for certain effector cells not regulated by *Fv-2*.

## 5 Effect of the *Fv-2* Gene on Normal and Malignant Hemopoietic (Erythroid) Cells

### 5.1 SFFV-Related Sequences and Friend Erythroleukemia Antigen in Hemopoietic Tissues

Recent studies indicate that sequences related to SFFV (the defective spleen focus forming component of the FV complex) are present in the DNA of normal mouse hemopoietic tissues, particularly in bone marrow and spleen (*Bernstein* et al. 1979). Such sequences are found in the DNA of both $Fv$-$2^{r/r}$ and $Fv$-$2^{s/s}$ mice. However, only in cells of $Fv$-$2^{s/s}$ mice are SFFV-related RNA sequences found. Studies with *Fv-2* congenic B6 ($Fv$-$2^{r/r}$) and B6.S ($Fv$-$2^{s/s}$) mice indicate that the $Fv$-$2^{s}$ allele regulates the presence of SFFV-related sequences in the RNA of spleen and bone marrow cells (*Mak* et al. 1979). Furthermore, when B6 and B6.S mice are infected with FV, high levels of SFFV-related RNA sequences are found only in spleen cells of B6.S mice. Thus the *Fv-2* locus seems to control both the expression of endogenous as well as exogenous SFFV-specific sequences. By utilizing an entirely different approach, Risser has found that hemopoietic tissues of normal and leukemic $Fv$-$2^{s/s}$ mice express a serologically detectable SFFV-specific cell surface antigen (called the FE antigen). Studies with congenic mice further demonstrate that the expression of FE antigen on normal hemopoietic cells is regulated by the *Fv-2* gene (*Risser* 1979). These findings have important implications, both with respect to normal hemopoiesis in mice as well as neoplastic transformation by FV. Conceivably, $Fv\text{-}2^{s/s}$ mice which express the SFFV-related sequences and FE antigen in their normal hemopoietic cells may be tolerant to such antigens. Therefore, they would fail to recognize and eliminate leukemic cells which express much larger amounts of the same antigen (*Risser* 1979). Since $Fv\text{-}2^{r/r}$ mice do possess SFFV-specific DNA sequences, their hemopoietic cells transformed by FV in vivo could express an FE-like antigen which would then be rapidly recognized by hosts not tolerant to the FE antigen. This conceivably could be the basis of $Fv\text{-}2$-mediated genetic resistance to FV leukemia. Whether immunocompetent cells other than T and B cells involved in the humoral antibody response to FE antigens can "recognize" FE antigens has not been determined. Certainly the role of M cells in regulating the response to FE needs to be examined. Another SFFV-specific antigen, defined serologically, has also been described. However, this antigen seems to be distinct from FE and its expression is not regulated by $Fv\text{-}2$ (*Yosook* et al. 1979).

## 5.2 $Fv\text{-}2$ and Cell Cycle Status of Burst Forming Units-Erythroid (BFU-E)

Another interesting and potentially important function of the $Fv\text{-}2$ gene appears to be the regulation of the cell-cycle status of primitive erythropoietic cells called burst forming units-erythroid (BFU-E). Axelrad and colleagues have found that a higher proportion of BFU-E in $Fv\text{-}2^{s/s}$ mice are engaged in DNA synthesis, whereas in $Fv\text{-}2^{r/r}$ mice the percentage of BFU-E in cycle is very low (*Suzuki* and *Axelrad* 1980). $F_1$ hybrid $Fv\text{-}2^{r/s}$ mice, which are susceptible to leukemia, also have a high proportion of their BFU-E in cell cycle. The allelic difference at the $Fv\text{-}2$ locus has no significant effect on other progenitor cells (i.e., colony forming unit-erythroid (CFU-E), colony forming unit-spleen (CFU-S). Procedures which cause hemopoietic cell regeneration in B6 mice also lead to an increase in the proportion of BFU-E in cycle. As compared with adults, B6 mice less than 4 weeks old also have a high percentage of BFU-E in cycle. On the basis of these findings, an argument could be made that $Fv\text{-}2$ regulates susceptibility to leukemia induction by regulating the numbers of BFU-E in cycle. It would follow that BFU-E in cycle are the target cells for transformation by FV. Studies in which partially congenic DBA/2. $Fv\text{-}2^r$ mice were tested suggested that one effect of $Fv\text{-}2^r$ gene is to inhibit SFFV replication (*Steeves* et al. 1978). This notion is consistent with the proposed role of $Fv\text{-}2$ in regulating the cell cycle status of BFU-E. In effect, such data support the target cell hypothesis for genetic resistance to FV. The loss of resistance in [89]Sr-treated B6 mice and the transformation of B10.D2 ($Fv\text{-}2^{r/r}$) bone marrow cells when transplanted into lethally irradiated leukemic DBA/2 ($Fv\text{-}2^{s/s}$) mice could be explained by assuming that such treatments increase the pool of BFU-E in cycle. If this is indeed the case, certain questions remain to be answered: how is the pool of BFU-E in cycle regulated in $Fv\text{-}2^{r/r}$ mice? Since M cells are known to be capable of regulating the growth of hemopoietic stem cells, could such cells regulate normal BFU-E and thus express $Fv\text{-}2$ function? Studies with [89]Sr-treated mice could answer this question. In the B10.D2 → DBA/2 transformation model (Sect. 2.2), transformed cells (TCFU) could be detected only during the first 2–3 weeks following transplantation of bone marrow cells into leukemic DBA/2 recipients (*Kumar* et al. 1974). Assuming that the B10.D2 cells underwent transformation due to an increase in cycling BFU-E under these conditions, what factors led to the arrest and elimination of the transformed $Fv-2^{r/r}$ cells after 3 weeks? It is interesting to note that the generation of new NK cells from their precursors in the bone marrow and the loss of B10.D2-transformed cells in the spleens of DBA/2 recipients both take about 2–3 weeks (*Kumar* et al. 1979b). It is quite likely that BFU-E are the target for transformation by Friend virus, and the cell cycle status of BFU-E may be a very important determinant in its susceptibility to transformation. Nevertheless, the mere availability of cycling BFU-E is unlikely to be the sole mechanism of genetic resistance against FV-induced erythroleukemia. Otherwise, almost any erythropoietic stress, e.g., bleeding, should abrogate $Fv-2^{r/r}$ resistance. Additional host defense mechanisms, mediated either by M cells and/or other immunocompetent cells, are also likely to be important.

## 6 Genetic Resistance to Immunesuppression

In susceptible mice, FV infection produces a rapid and profound immunosuppression, predominantly of humoral immunity. The mechanism of FV-induced suppression of the anti-SRBC plaque-forming response has been extensively investigated (*Bennett* and *Steeves* 1970; *Ceglowski* and *Friedman* 1969; *Ceglowski* 1975; *Cerny* and *Waner* 1975; *Cerny* et al. 1976). Infection with FV affects early stages of B cell differentiation; T helper cells are unaffected. Accessory cells have been reported as normal or deficient in function (*Bendinelli* et al. 1976). Mice genetically resistant to the leukemogenic effect of FV are also relatively resistant to the immunosuppressive effects of FV (*Ceglowski* and *Friedman* 1969; *Kumar* et al. 1978a, b). The immunosuppression produced by FV inoculation in such mice is mild and transient. However, when genetically resistant C57BL/6 mice were treated with [89]Sr and then inoculated with FV, not only did they show malignant erythroblastosis, but the anti-SRBC response was also profoundly suppressed (*Kumar* et al. 1974).

## 6.1 Genetic Resistance to Suppression of Lymphocyte Mitogenesis

To analyze the mechanism of genetic resistance to immunosuppression and its abrogation in [89]Sr-treated mice, an in vitro approach was adopted (*Kumar* and *Bennett* 1976). Mitogenesis of lymphoid cells obtained from mice susceptible to FV leukemia is markedly suppressed in the presence of FV in culture. FV induces suppression of both B-cell and T-cell mitogenesis obtained from spleen, lymph nodes, thymus, and bone marrow of susceptible mice. However, the mitogenesis of lymphoid cells obtained from genetically resistant mice is much less affected by similar doses of FV in vitro (Table 3). This difference in the in vitro susceptibility/resistance to the suppressive effect of FV is not affected by genes within the *H-2* complex. Unlike spleen cells from normal B6 mice, however, Con A-induced mitogenesis of spleen cells from [89]Sr-treated mice was markedly suppressed (*Kumar* and *Bennett* 1976). A major question which arose from such a study was: Does treatment of mice with [89]Sr alter their mitogen-responsive T and B cells, or is the susceptibility to the suppression of mitogen response mediated indirectly? To answer this question, an understanding of the mechanisms by which FV suppresses the lymphocyte mitogenesis of leukemia susceptible mice is discussed first.

Table 3. Strain distribution of susceptibility to FV-induced suppression of mitogenic response of T and B cells[a]

| Experiment | Mouse strain[a] | H-2 type | Lymphoid cell source | Mitogen | Percent suppression of mitogenesis by FV |
|---|---|---|---|---|---|
| 1 | DBA/2 | d | Spleen | Con A[b] | 84 |
|   | B10.D2/n | d | Spleen | Con A | 13[e] |
| 2 | 129 | b | Thymus | Con A | 78 |
|   | B6 | b | Thymus | Con A | -18[e] |
| 3 | C3H | k | Spleen | Con A | 58 |
|   | C58 | k | Spleen | Con A | 4[e] |
| 4 | 129 | b | Spleen | LPS[c] | 68 |
|   | B6 | b | Spleen | LPS | 22 |
| 5 | DBA/2 | d | Spleen | LPS | 75 |
|   | B10.D2 | d | Spleen | LPS | 29 |
| 6 | 129 | b | Bone marrow | DS[d] | 85 |
|   | B6 | b | Bone marrow | DS | 7[e] |
| 7 | DBA/2 | d | Bone marrow | DS | 58 |
|   | B10.D2 | d | Bone marrow | DS | 9[e] |

Modified from *Kumar* and *Bennett* 1976
[a] DBA/2, 129, and C3H mice are susceptible to FV leukemia in vivo. DBA/2, 129, C3H, and C58 mice possess the $Fv-1^n$ genotype. The rest, i.e., B10.D2 and B6, are $Fv-1^b$
[b] Con A = Concanavalin A
[c] LPS = Lipopolysaccharide
[d] DS = Dextran sulfate
[e] Not significantly different from control (no FV) value ($P > 0.05$). Suppression of $\Delta$ blastogenesis was significantly greater ($P < 0.05$ as determined by Student's $t$-test) in cells from susceptible donors in each experiment

## 6.2 Suppression of Lymphocyte Mitogenesis – Mechanisms

Suppression of lymphocyte mitogenesis by FV could either be a direct effect on the responding cells or, alternately, be mediated by suppressor cells. Depletion of macrophages and B cells from the spleen of susceptible BALB/c and C3H mice fails to alter their susceptibility to FV-induced suppression of mitogenesis. However, following filtration of spleen cells over nylon wool, the Con A-induced mitogenesis is no longer suppressed by FV. Addition of normal +/+ spleen cells to the nylon-filtered cells restores their susceptibility to FV in vitro. On the other hand, addition of normal spleen cells from *nu/nu* donors to the nylon-filtered spleen cell population failed to restore susceptibility to the effects of FV in vitro (Table 4). These and other experiments suggest that FV-induced suppression of lectin-induced T-cell mitogenesis in vitro is mediated by T suppressor cells (TSC), which are nylon wool adherent and are absent from the spleens of athymic nude mice (*Kumar* et al. 1976). TSC which are activated by FV to cause suppression of mitogen-responsive T and B cells are weakly Thyl. 2 positive and are present in the normal spleen as well as thymus. In the thymus TSC belong to the cortisol-sensitive population. Spleen cells of genetically resistant mice are not intrinsically resistant to the

Table 4. Effect of FV on the suppression of Con A-induced mitogenesis of BAlB/c lymphocytes[a]

| Experiment | Source of cells stimulated by Con A | Percent suppression of mitogenesis by FV |
|---|---|---|
| 1 | Whole spleen (W) | 62 |
|   | Nylon wool filtered (NF) | 9 |
|   | NF + W (1:1) | 56 |
| 2 | W | 55 |
|   | NF | 7 |
|   | NF + W (5:1) | 52 |
|   | NF + W (10:1) | 54 |
|   | NF + W (15:1) | 37 |
| 3 | W *(nu/+)* | 48 |
|   | NF *(nu/+)* | 8 |
|   | NF *(nu/+)* + W *(nu/+)* (10:1) | 56 |
|   | NF *(nu/+)* + W *(nu/nu)* (10:1) | 8 |

Modified from *Kumar* et al. 1976

[a] NF spleen cells were less suppressible ($P < 0.05$) than whole spleen cells (exps. 1–3). NF + W mixture of spleen cells were significantly ($P < 0.05$) more suppressed than spleen cells (exps. 1–3), except in exp. 3 when *nu/nu* W spleen cells were used

suppressive effects of FV, but lack TSC function. In support of this is the finding that when spleen cells from leukemia-resistant B10.D2 ($H$-$2^d$, $Fv$-$2^{r/r}$) mice and leukemia-susceptible DBA/2 ($H$-$2^d$, $Fv$-$2^{s/s}$) are mixed in a ratio of 9:1 and then tested in vitro, the mitogen responsive cells of the B10.D2 mice are fully susceptible to the suppressive effects of FV. The source of TSC in such a mixture is DBA/2 spleen cells, which can be irradiated (1000 R) in vitro to prevent their proliferation. Interestingly, such mixture experiments indicated that TSCs which are activated by FV to suppress MRC must share the D end of $H$-$2$ (*Kumar* and *Bennett* 1977).

## 6.3 Suppression of Lymphocyte Mitogenesis: the *Fv-3* Gene

The in vitro model involving stimulation of lymphocyte mitogenesis in the presence or absence of FV reflects the in vivo susceptibility/resistance to the immunosuppressive effects of FV on antibody synthesis. Since mice which are susceptible to spleen focus forming virus in vivo, i.e., $Fv$-$2^{s/s}$, are also susceptible to immunosuppressive effects of FV both in vivo and in vitro and $Fv$-$2^{r/r}$ mice are resistant to the immunosuppression by FV, $Fv$-$2$ could be the locus which regulates the susceptibility to immunosuppression. However, experiments designed to test this point directly indicated that susceptibility to immunosuppression is under separate genetic control. DBA/2 ($H$-$2^d$, $Fv$-$2^{s/s}$), B10.D2 ($H$-$2^d$, $Fv$-$2^{r/r}$), (DBA/2 X B10.D2) $F_1$, $F_2$, and backcross mice were hemisplenectomized and typed for susceptibility to immunosuppression by FV in vitro. Subsequently the same mice were typed for $Fv$-$2$ by injecting them with FV. Similar typing for $Fv$-$2$ and susceptibility to immunosuppression in vitro was also performed by utilizing the $F_2$ progeny of 129 ($Fv$-$2^{s/s}$, $H$-$2^b$) and B6 ($Fv$-$2^{r/r}$, $H$-$2^b$) mice. Results from such experiments clearly indicated that susceptibility to immunosuppression in vitro and to spleen focus formation

Table 5. Typing of individual (DBA/2 X B10.D2) X B10.D2 backcross mice for susceptibility to spleen focus formation in vivo and suppression of Con A-induced lymphocyte mitogenesis in vitro[a]

| Mice | Susceptibility to spleen focus formation | Percent suppression of mitogenesis by FV |
|------|------------------------------------------|------------------------------------------|
| | | Mean $\pm$ SEM |
| B10.D2 | – | $2 \pm 13.8$ |
| DBA/2 | + | $68.7 \pm 2.7$ |
| | | Individual values |
| Backcross progeny (12) | + | –5, 5, 15, 15, 16, 42, 43, 61, 62, 62, 80 |
| Backcross progeny (8) | – | –30, –5, 0, 20, 40, 45, 50, 85 |

[a] No correlation between susceptibility to spleen focus formation and susceptibility to suppression of T cell mitogenesis by Friend virus (FV)

(Fv-2 effect) in vivo segregated independently (Table 5). The susceptibility to immunosuppression in vitro is regulated by a single gene, dominant for susceptibility, called Fv-3 (Kumar et al. 1978a). Fv-3 is not linked to H-2, and most mice sharing the C57BL/6 background are Fv-3$^{r/r}$. Since such mice also possess immune-response (IC)-like genes which confer upon them "good responder status" against grafts of incompatible H-2$^{d}$ bone marrow cells, we also investigated the possible linkage of Fv-3 to genes which regulate the anti-Hh response against H-2$^{d}$ bone marrow allografts. These studies indicated that Fv-3 segregated independently of such Ir-like genes (Kumar et al. 1978a). Not only does Fv-3 regulate susceptibility to suppression of lymphocyte mitogenesis in vitro, but it also regulates the genetic susceptibility to suppression of humoral antibody forming cells in vivo. This conclusion is derived from experiments in which (B10.D2 X DBA/2) F$_1$ mice backcrossed to the B10.D2 parent were individually typed for Fv-3 by in vitro lymphocyte mitogenesis assay and suppression of anti-SRBC plaque-forming cell response in vivo (Kumar et al. 1978b). A very good concordance between susceptibility to immunosuppression in vivo and in vitro was seen.

## 6.4 Mechanism of Fv-3 Gene Function

Since Fv-3$^{s/s}$ mice possess TSC, which mediate the immunosuppressive effect of FV, and Fv-3$^{r/r}$ mice are lacking in such TSC function, it follows that Fv-3 may act by regulating either the function and/or numbers of suppressor cells which are "activated" by FV. How may such a regulation occur? As mentioned earlier, Fv-3$^{r/r}$ mice become susceptible to the immunosuppressive effect of FV both in vivo and in vitro following treatment with $^{89}$Sr. Cell mixture and nylon wool filtration experiments indicate that the susceptibility of $^{89}$Sr-treated Fv-3$^{r/r}$ mice results from acquisition of T suppressor cell function similar to that which is normally seen in Fv-3$^{s/s}$ mice (Table 6). This data suggest that Fv-3$^{r/r}$ may mediate its regulatory role on TSC via M cells. It is not clear how Fv-3 may govern M cell-TSC interaction. Two possible mechanisms may be suggested. First, Fv-3 could affect the antigenicity of suppressor cells such that they are recognized and eliminated by M cells. Alternatively, Fv-3 may affect the ability of M cells to recognize and/or interact with TSC.

Table 6. Effect of FV on Con A-induced mitogenesis of spleen cells from normal and [89]Sr-treated C57BL/6 mice[a]

| Experiment | Mouse pretreatment | Percent suppression of mitogenesis by FV |
|---|---|---|
| 1 | None (control) | 7[b] |
|  | [89]Sr | 42 |
|  | [89]Sr (NF)[c] | – 4[b] |
| 2 | None (control) | 5[b] |
|  | [89]Sr | 60 |
|  | 3:1 Control: [89]Sr spleen cells[c] | 55 |
|  | 9:1 Control: [89]Sr spleen cells[c] | 48 |

Modified from *Kumar* et al. 1976
[a] Whole spleen cells from B6 mice treated with [89]Sr were significantly more suppressible than whole spleen cells from control B6 mice or NF spleen cells from [89]Sr-treated B6 mice (exp. 1). Mixtures of spleen cells from control and [89]Sr-treated B6 mice were significantly ($P<0.05$) more suppressible than spleen cells from control B6 mice (exp. 2). FV = Friend virus; NF = nylon Filtered
[b] Not significantly different from control (no FV)
[c] Spleen cells from [89]Sr-treated and control B6 mice were mixed in the ratios indicated before culture

Administration of [89]Sr to mice results not only in the generation of functional TSC in the FV system but also in several other models. [89]Sr-treated mice possess suppressor cells which in the presence of suitable activating stimuli can suppress antibody forming cells, certain cytotoxic T cell precursors, and those NK cells whose functional activity is normal in [89]Sr-treated mice, e.g., NK (EL-4) (*Merluzzi* et al. 1978; *Luevano* et al., to be published). It is conceivable that the generation of suppressor cell activity in [89]Sr-treated mice results merely from a shift of hematopoiesis to the spleen. Alternatively, M cells may have an important regulatory influence on the function of suppressor cells. The finding of an NK-sensitive population within the thymus of infant mice raises some interesting possibilities in this respect (*Hansson* et al. 1979). NK-sensitive thymocytes of A-strain mice seem to express determinants similar to those expressed by YAC-1 tumor cells. [89]Sr-treated B6D2 F$_1$ mice, which are deficient in M cell (NK-YAC-1) function, are also unable to lyse NK-sensitive thymocytes from A-strain mice (*Kumar, Kornfeld* and *Bennett*, unpublished work). The presence of NK-sensitive thymocytes seems to be inversely related to the M-cell status of the mice. It is conceivable that M cells regulate T suppressor cells by the recognition of certain differentiation-specific antigens present on TSC. Such a link in M cell-TSC interaction would be strengthened if the NK-sensitive thymocytes possess functional properties of TSC. This interesting possibility remains to be explored.

# 7 Conclusions

Treatment of mice by the bone-seeking isotope [89]Sr has a profound effect on their genetic resistance to FV-induced leukemogenesis and immunosuppression. While the mechanisms of this effect of $^{89}$Sr are not entirely clear, it is suggested that they are mediated by the abrogation of M cell functions. NK activity against YAC-1 lymphoma cells seems to fulfill several criteria for an in vitro analogue of M cells. In the uninfected animal, M cells may have an immunoregulatory function expressed at the level of suppressor cells available for activation by FV (*Fv-3* gene effect). Mice of the genotype *Fv-3$^{r/r}$* lack such suppressor cell function and hence are largely protected from the immunosuppressive effects of FV. Following infection with FV, resistance to leukemogenesis, which is a function of the *Fv-2* gene, may involve recognition and elimination of transformed erythroid target cells by marrow-dependent effector cells. The *Fv-2* gene is clearly the major determinant of the induction of leukemia, since in mice segregating for *Fv-2* and *Fv-3* genes, the resistance to leukemia induction conferred by the *Fv-2$^{r/r}$* genotype cannot be overriden by the presence of *Fv-3$^{s/s}$* alleles. Conversely, *Fv-3$^{r/r}$* mice in the segregating population are not protected from leukemia induction if they have the genotype *Fv-2$^{r/s}$*. The *Fv-3* gene may therefore mediate its protective effects, if any, by regulating events which take place after leukemia induction, i.e., progression/regression of the disease. Although *Fv-3* is distinct from the *Rfv* genes, such genes may together regulate the genetic ability to recover from the leukemia.

*Acknowledgments.* Research described in this review is supported by grants CA-21401, CA-15369, and HL-24201 from the National Institutes of Health, and grant IM-29 from the American Cancer Society. V.K. is recipient of a Cancer Research Scholar Award from the American Cancer Society (Mass. Div). The assistance of *Mary Carol Barnes* in the preparation of this manuscript is greatly appreciated.

# References

Axelrad AA, Steeves RA (1964) Assay for Friend virus: rapid quantification method based on enumeration of macroscopic spleen foci in mice. Virology 24:513

Axelrad A, Gaag HC van der (1968) Genetic and cellular basis of susceptibility or resistance to Friend leukemia virus infection in mice. Canadian Cancer Conf 8:313

Bendinelli M, Toniolo A, Friedman H (1976) Reversal of immunosuppression induced by murine leukemia viruses. Ann NY Acad Sci 276:431

Bennett M (1972) Marrow allograft rejection: importance of *H-2* homozygosity of donor cells. Transplantation 14:289

Bennett M (1973) Prevention of marrow allograft rejection with radioactive strontium: evidence for marrow dependent effector cells. J Immunol 110:510

Bennett M, Eckner RJ (1973) Immunobiology of Friend virus leukemia. In: Ceglowski WS, Friedman H (eds) Virus tumorigenesis and immunogenesis. Academic Press, New York, p 387

Bennett M, Steeves RA (1970) Immunocompetent cell functions in mice infected with Friend leukemia virus. J Natl Cancer Inst 44:1107

Bennett M, Baker EE, Eastcott JW, Kumar V, Yonkosky D (1976) Selective elimination of marrow precursors with the bone seeking isotope $^{89}$Sr: implication for hemopoiesis, lymphopoiesis, viral leukemogenesis and infection. J Reticuloendothel Soc 20:71

Bennett M, Kumar V, Levy EM, Rodday P (1980) Genetic resistance to tumors: role of marrow dependent and independent cells. In: Skamene E, Kongshavn PAL, Landy M (eds) Genetic control of natural resistance to infection and malignancy. Academic Press, New York, p 431–443

Bernstein A, Gamble CL, Penrose D, Mak TW (1979) Presence and expression of Friend erythroleukemia virus-related sequences in normal and leukemic mouse tissue. Proc Natl Acad Sci USA 76:4455–4459

Burton RC, Bartlett SP, Kumar V, Winn H (1981) Heterogeneity of natural killer cells in the mouse. Transpl Proc XIII:783–786

Ceglowski WS (1975) Effect of leukemia virus infection on antibody formation and cellular immunity. Ann NY Acad Sci 276:411

Ceglowski WS, Friedman H (1969) Murine virus leukemogenesis: relationship between susceptibility and immunodepression. Nature 224:1318

Cerny J, Waner EB (1975) Specific susceptibility of sensitized (memory) B cells to suppression and antigenic alteration by murine leukemia virus. J Immunol 114:571

Cerny J, Hensgen PA, Fistel SF, Mastalir-Demler L (1976) Interaction of murine leukemia virus with isolated lymphocytes. II. Infection of B and T cells with Friend virus complex in vitro: effect of polyclonal mitogens. Int J Cancer 18:189

Chesebro B, Wehrly K (1978) *Rfv-1* and *Rfv-2*, two *H-2* associated genes that influence recovery from Friend leukemia virus induced splenomegaly. J Immunol 120:1081–1085

Chesebro B, Wehrly K (1979) Identification of a non-*H-2* gene (*Rfv-3*) influencing recovery from viremia and leukemia induced by Friend virus complex. Proc Natl Acad Sci USA 76:425–429

Chesebro B, Wehrly K, Stimpfling JH (1974) Host genetic control of recovery from Friend leukemia virus-induced splenomegaly. Mapping of a gene within the major histocompatibility complex. J Exp Med 140:1457

Cudkowicz G (1971) Genetic control of bone marrow graft rejection. I. Determinant specific difference of reactivity in two pairs of inbred mice strains. J Exp Med 134:281

Cudkowicz G, Bennett M (1971a) Peculiar immunobiology of bone marrow allografts. I. Graft rejection by irradiated responder mice. J Exp Med 134:83

Cudkowicz G, Bennett M (1971b) Peculiar immunobiology of bone marrow allografts. II. Rejection of parental grafts by resistant F₁ hybrid mice. J Exp Med 134:1513

Cudkowicz G, Hochman PS (1979) Do natural killer cells engage in regulated reaction against self to ensure homeostasis. Immunol Rev 44:13

Cudkowicz G, Yung YP (1977) Abrogation of resistance to foreign bone marrow grafts by carrageenans. I. Studies with the antimacrophage agent, Seakem carrageenan. J Immunol 119:483

Fitzgerald PA, Bennett M (submitted) Aging and [89]Sr-treated mice: loss of responsiveness to syngeneic but not to allogeneic cells

Fried W, Gurney CW, Swatek M (1966) Effect of Strontium-89 on the stem cell compartment of the spleen. Radiat Res 29:50

Furmanski P, Dietz M, Fouchey S, Hall L, Clyme R, Rich MA (1979) Spontaneous regression of Friend murine leukemia virus induced erythroleukemia. IV. Effect of radiation and athymia on leukemia regression in mice. J Natl Cancer Inst 63:449–454

Gurney CW, Klassen L, Birks J, Allen E (1972) Hematopoietic and immunologic alterations in mice produced by [89]Sr-induced marrow hypoplasia. Exp Hematol 22:27

Haller O, Wigzell H (1977) Suppression of natural killer cell activity with radioactive strontium: effector cells are marrow-dependent. J Immunol 118:1503

Haller O, Kiessling R, Orn A, Wigzell H (1977) Generation of natural killer cells: a autonomous function of bone marrow. J Exp Med 145:1411

Hansson M, Kärre K, Kiessling R, Roder J, Andersson B, Häyry P (1979) Natural NK cell targets in the mouse thymus: characteristics of the sensitive cell population. J Immunol 123:765

Hochman PS, Cudkowicz G (1977) Different sensitivities to hydrocortisone of natural killer cell activity and hybrid resistance to parental bone marrow grafts. J Immunol 119:2013–2015

Kiessling R, Hochman PS, Haller O, Shearer GM, Wigzell H, Cudkowicz G (1977) Evidence for a similar or common mechanism for natural killer activity and resistance to hemopoietic grafts. Eur J Immunol 7:655

Kumar V, Bennett M (1976) Mechanisms of genetic resistance to Friend virus leukemia in mice. II. Resistance of mitogen-responsive cells mediated by marrow-dependent cells. J Exp Med 143:713

Kumar V, Bennett M (1977) *H-2* compatibility requirements for T-suppressor cell functions induced by Friend leukemia virus. Nature 265:345

Kumar V, Bennett M, Eckner RJ (1974) Mechanism of genetic resistance to Friend virus leukemia in mice. I. Role of [89]Sr-sensitive effector cells responsible for rejection of marrow allografts. J Exp Med 139:1093

Kumar V, Caruso T, Bennett M (1976) Mechanism of genetic resistance to Friend virus leukemia. III. Susceptibility of mitogen responsive lymphocytes mediated by T cells. J Exp Med 143:728

Kumar V, Goldschmidt L, Eastcott JW, Bennett M (1978a) Mechanism of genetic resistance to

Friend virus leukemia in mice. IV. Identification of a gene (*Fv-3*) regulating immunosuppression in vitro, and its distinction from *Fv-2* and genes regulating marrow allograft reactivity. J Exp Med 147:422

Kumar V, Resnick P, Eastcott JW, Bennett M (1978b) Mechanism of genetic resistance to Friend virus leukemia in mice. V. Relevance of *Fv-3* gene in the regulation of in vivo immunosuppression. J Natl Cancer Inst 61:1117–1123

Kumar V, Leuvano E, Bennett M (1979a) Hybrid resistance to EL-4 lymphoma cells. I. Characterization of natural killer cells which lyse EL-4 cells and their distinction from marrow-dependent natural killer cell. J Exp Med 150:531

Kumar V, Ben-Ezra J, Bennett M, Sonnenfeld G (1979b) Natural killer cells in mice treated with [89]Strontium: normal target binding cell numbers but inability to kill even after interferon administration. J Immunol 123:1832

Levy EA, Kumar V, Bennett M (1980) Interaction between spleen cells from normal and [89]Sr-treated mice upon adoptive transfer. Fed Proc 39:671

Lilly F (1970) *Fv-2*: identification and location of a second gene governing the spleen focus response to Friend leukemia virus in mice. J Natl Cancer Inst 45:163

Luevano E, Kumar V, Bennett M (to be published) Hybrid resistance to EL-4 lymphoma cells. II. Association between loss of hybrid resistance with detection of suppressor cells after treatment of mice with [89]Sr. Scand J Immunol

Lotzova E (1977) Involvement of MHC-linked hemopoietic histocompatibility genes in allogeneic bone marrow transplantation in mice. Tissue Antigens 9:148

Lotzova E, Cudkowicz G (1974) Abrogation of resistance to bone marrow grafts by silica particles. Prevention of silica effect by the macrophage stabilizer poly-2-vinylpyridine-N-oxide. J Immunol 113:798

Lust JA, Kumar V, Bennett M (1980) Friend virus induced erythroleukemia cells (FLD-3): rejection by irradiated mice and lysis by Natural Killer cells. Fed Proc 39:1150

Mak T, Axelrad A, Bernstein A (1979) The *Fv-2* locus controls expression of Friend erythroleukemia virus specific sequences in normal and infected mice. Proc Natl Acad Sci USA 76:5809–5812

Manning DD, Koultab NM, Jutilla JW (1974) Effect of anti-mu-specific immunosuppression on Friend virus leukemia. J Immunol 112:1698–1704

Masuda A, Bennett M (to be published) Concanavalin A induced resistance to *Listeria monocytogenes* (LM): defect in mice treated with radioactive strontium. Eur J Immunol

Merluzzi VJ, Levy EM, Kumar V, Bennett M, Cooperband SR (1978) In vitro activation of suppressor cells from spleens of mice treated with radioactive strontium. J Immunol 121:505

Mirand EA, Steeves RA, Avila L, Grace Jr JT (1968) Spleen focus formation by polycythemic strains of Friend leukemia virus. Proc Soc Exp Bio Med 127:900

Mortensen RF, Ceglowski WS, Friedman H (1974) Leukemia virus-induced immunosuppression. X. Depression of T cell mediated cytotoxicity after infection of mice with Friend leukemia virus. J Immunol 112:2077

Odaka T, Matsukura M (1969) Inheritance of susceptibility to Friend mouse leukemia virus. VI. Reciprocal alterations of innate resistance or susceptibility by bone marrow transplantation between congenic strains. J Virol 4:837

Ojo E, Wigzell H (1978) Natural killer cells may be the only cells in normal mouse lymphoid cell populations endowed with cytotoxic ability for antibody coated tumor target cells. Scand J Immunol 7:297

Pincus T, Rowe WP, Lilly F (1971) A major genetic locus affecting resistance to infection with murine leukemia viruses. II. Apparent identity to a major locus described for resistance to Friend murine leukemia virus. J Exp Med 133:1234

Risser R (1979) Friend erythroleukemia antigen: a viral antigen specified by spleen focus forming virus (SFFV) and differentiation antigen controlled by *Fv-2*. J Exp Med 149:1152–1167

Rossi GB, Cudkowicz G, Friend C (1973) Transformation of spleen cells three hours after infection in vivo with Friend leukemia virus. J Natl Cancer Inst 50:249

Santoni A, Herberman RB, Holden HT (1979) Correlation between natural and antibody-dependent cell mediated cytotoxicity against tumor cells in mouse. I. Distribution of the reactivity. J Natl Cancer Inst 62:109

Seaman WE, Gindhart TD, Greenspan JS, Blackman MA, Talal N (1979) Natural killer cells, bone and the bone-marrow: studies in estrogen treated mice and congenitally osteopetrotic *(mi/mi)* mice. J Immunol 122:2541

Steeves RA, Eckner RJ, Bennett M, Mirand EA (1971) Isolation and characterization of a lymphatic leukemia virus in the Friend virus complex. J Natl Cancer Inst 46:1209

Steeves RA, Lilly F, Steinheider G, Blank KJ (1978) The effect of the *Fv-2ʳ* gene on spleen focus forming virus and embryonic development. In: Clarkson B, Marks PA, Till JE (eds) Differentiation of normal and neoplastic hematopoietic cells. Cold Spring Harbor Laboratory, p 591

Stutman O, Dupuy J (1972) Resistance to Friend leukemia virus in mice: effect of immunosuppression. J Natl Cancer Inst 49:1283

Suzuki S, Axelrad A (1980) *Fv-2* locus controls the proportion of erythropoietic progenitor cells (BFU-E) synthesizing DNA in normal mice. Cell 19:225–236

Troxler DH, Parks WP, Vaas WC, Scolnick EM (1977) Isolation of a fibroblast non-producer cell line containing the Friend strain of the spleen focus forming virus. Virology 76:615

Yoosook C, Steeves RA, Ruscetti S (1979) Specific neutralization of defective spleen focus forming virus in Friend virus complex by rat antiserum. J Virol 31:408–414

# Natural Cell-Mediated Immunity During Viral Infections

RAYMOND M. WELSH*

## 1 Introduction

Viral infections elicit both specific and nonspecific responses in infected hosts. The specific responses include the production of antiviral antibody and the generation of virus-specific cytotoxic T cells. The non-specific responses include the elevation of body temperature, the synthesis of interferon, and the activation of macrophages and natural killer (NK) cells. While most of these parameters have been studied for a number of years, only recently has the concept been proposed that NK cells may contribute to the resistance or pathology in viral infections (reviewed in *Welsh* 1978a). This concept is par-

*University of Massachusetts Medical Center, 55 Lake Avenue North, Worcester, Massachusetts
 01605, USA

ticularly intriguing because NK cells may have the capacity to mediate both nonspecific and specific arms of the host response. Many investigators agree that NK cells and K lymphocytes, mediators of antibody-dependent, cell mediated cytotoxicity (ADCC), may represent identical, overlapping, or similar populations of effector cells (*Ojo* and *Wigzell* 1978; *Herberman* et al. 1979; *Pape* et al. 1979; *Timonen* 1979).

NK or NK-like cells have been found in virtually every mammalian species examined and even in invertebrates. However, this review will mostly discuss work on human and mouse NK cells, which have been the most extensively studied. For reviews on the properties of NK cells, see *Kiessling* and *Wigzell* (1979) and *Herberman* et al. (1979). Human NK cells are lymphocytes possessing low affinity receptors for sheep erythrocytes and high-affinity receptors for the Fc region of human immunoglubulin G (IgG). They are not phagocytic or plastic adherent and do not bear significant levels or surface Ig. Mouse NK cells express low levels of theta antigen and low affinity Fc receptors for IgG. Like the human NK cells, they are not phagocytic or plastic adherent and do not have detectable levels of surface Ig. Recently, other markers have been obtained which distinguish mouse NK cells from cytotoxic T cells and other lymphocytes. Mouse NK activity can be preferentially depleted by treatment of spleen leukocytes with complement and antiserum directed against Ly 5 (*Kasai* et al. 1979), NK antigen (*Glimcher* et al. 1977), and asialo-GM-1, a neutral glycolipid (*Young* et al. 1980). Mouse NK cell activity is low at birth, rises to a peak at 4 to 10 weeks of age, and thereafter gradually declines with age (*Kiessling* et al. 1975a; *Herberman* et al. 1975). NK cell development is independent of the thymus but dependent on the integrity of the bone marrow, i.e., athymic nude mice have normal or higher than normal levels of NK cells, while mice treated with antiserum to bone marrow or with $^{89}$Sr, an analog of calcium which deposits in the bone marrow, have very low levels of NK activity (*Haller* and *Wigzell* 1977; *Haller* et al. 1977).

Human and mouse NK cell activity is normally directed against a limited number of tumor target cells. However, the activity of NK cells can be greatly augmented by interferon (*Trinchieri* and *Santoli* 1978; *Gidlund* et al. 1978; *Welsh* 1978b), and these resulting activated NK cells can then lyse nearly any type of target cell to which they are exposed. It is the property of virus infections to induce interferon which in turn can activate NK cells that renders the role of NK cells in virus infections a particularly important question to resolve.

## 2 Induction of NK Cell Activity by Virus Infection in Vivo

### 2.1 Historical

Most work on the induction of NK cell activity in vivo by virus infections has been done in the mouse model. To put things in perspective, virus-induced lymphocyte killing of virus-infected cells was first reported in 1969 by *Lundstedt* (1969), who used the lymphocytic choriomeningitis virus (LCMV) system. After a series of elegant cell transfer studies which established a role for theta-bearing (T) cells in the pathology of LCMV-infected mice (*Cole* et al. 1972; *Gilden* et al. 1972), Cole and co-workers showed that T lymphocytes mediated virus-specific cell cytotoxicity in vitro (*Cole* et al. 1973). Soon thereafter, *Zinkernagel* and *Doherty* (1974) reported their very interesting discovery that the T cell killing in the LCMV system was not only virus specific but was also restricted to target cells bearing histocompatibility antigens syngeneic with the effector cells. Concurrently, several laboratories reported the first descriptions of naturally occurring cytotoxic lymphocytes which lysed in vitro certain types of tumor cells, particularly T-cell lymphomas (*Kiessling* et al. 1975b; *Herberman* et al. 1973; *Zarling* et al. 1975). All groups agreed that these cells, termed natural killer (NK) cells by *Kiessling* et al. (1975a, b), were nonadherent to nylon wool and insensitive to anti-theta antiserum and complement.

Undoubtedly, the early investigators of virus-specific T cell killing must have encountered some NK cell-mediated lysis in their assays as well. *Pfizenmaier* et al. (1975), working with LCMV, and *Blanden* and *Gardner* (1976), working with ectromelia, each reported the induction of non-virus-specific cytotoxic T cells peaking shortly before the specific T-cell response. *Rodda* and *White* (1976) examined "nonspecific" cytotoxic peritoneal cells of mice induced in the early stages of the Semliki forest virus infection and concluded that the effector cells were cytotoxic macrophages. Those reports were written before the existence and ubiquity of NK cells were widely recognized, and it is probable that the cytotoxic cells in question were actually NK cells. As we shall discuss later, activated NK cells may express enhanced adherence properties, making them confusable with macrophages, and anti-theta sensitivity, rendering them confusable with T cells.

In 1977 several groups reported that NK cell activity was greatly augmented during

Table 1. Activation of NK cells by virus infections in Vivo

| Virus | Host | References |
|---|---|---|
| Adeno | Mouse | *Herberman* et al. 1977 |
| Cytomegalo | Mouse | *Quinnan* and *Manischewitz* 1977[a] |
| Coxsackie | Mouse | *Wong* et al. 1977[a] |
| Ectromelia | Mouse | *Blanden* and *Gardner* 1976? |
| Gross C-type | Mouse | *Herberman* et al. 1977 |
| Kilham rat | Rat | *Oehler* et al. 1978 |
| Kunjin | Mouse | *MacFarlan* et al. 1977[a] |
| Lactic dehydrogenase | Mouse | *Herberman* et al. 1977 |
| Lymphocytic choriomeningitis | Mouse | *Herberman* et al. 1977; *Welsh* and *Zinkernagel* 1977[a]; *Welsh* 1978[a] |
| Lymphocytic choriomeningitis | Rat | *Oehler* et al. 1978 |
| Mumps | Mouse | *Minato* et al. 1979 |
| Minute virus of mice | Mouse | *Herberman* et al. 1977 |
| Moloney sarcoma | Mouse | *Herberman* et al. 1977 |
| Mouse hepatitis | Mouse | *Herberman* et al. 1977 |
| Mouse salivary gland | Mouse | *Herberman* et al. 1977 |
| Newcastle disease | Mouse | *Gidlund* et al. 1978 |
| Pichinde | Hamster | *Gee* et al. 1980[a] |
| Pichinde | Mouse | *Welsh* 1978 |
| Polyoma | Mouse | *Herberman* et al. 1977 |
| Semliki forest | Mouse | *MacFarlan* et al. 1977 |
| Vaccinia | Mouse | *Welsh* et al. 1979 |
| Vesicular stomatitis | Mouse | *Minato* et al. 1979 |
| Xenotropic C-type | Mouse | *Herberman* et al. 1977 |

[a] Denote papers which have characterized the cells induced by the specific virus in question. The question mark refers to a study in which the cells were characterized but concluded at that time to be T cells

virus infections in mice (*Herberman* et al. 1977; *MacFarlan* et al. 1977; *Welsh* and *Zinkernagel* 1977). Similar NK-cell augmentation was subsequently found in other species as well (Table 1). The effector cells induced by only a few of those viruses have been characterized, with the most extensive work done in the LCMV (*Welsh* and *Zinkernagel* 1977; *Welsh* 1978b; *Tai* et al. 1980; *Kiessling* et al. 1980) and Kunjin virus (*MacFarlan* et al. 1977, 1979) systems. While this review will emphasize our work on the LCMV infection, it should be pointed out that work from other groups with different viruses has led to some of the same conclusions (*MacFarlan* et al. 1977, 1979; *Quinnan* and *Manischewitz* 1979).

## 2.2 Induction of NK Cell Activity and Association with Interferon Synthesis

The LCMV infection of mice results in the generation of two peaks of cytotoxic spleen leukocytes (Fig. 1). The level of activity and the day of appearance of each peak can be shifted, depending on the dose of virus given. The first peak contains activated NK cells, while the second peak harbors the virus-specific cytotoxic T cells *(Welsh* and *Zinkernagel* 1977; *Welsh* 1978b). The induction of NK cell activity in LCMV-infected mice directly parallels the levels of virus-induced interferon, as shown in Figure 2 (*Welsh* 1978b). Injection of mice intraperitoneally (*Welsh* 1978b) or intravenously (*Gidlund* et al. 1978) with fibroblast interferon type I or intraperitoneally (*Kumar* et al. 1979a) with interferon type II also results in NK cell activation. Treatment of mice infected with Newcastle disease virus (NDV) with antibody to mouse fibroblast interferon prevented the augmentation of NK cell activity, confirming the hypothesis that virus-induced interferon activates NK cells in vivo (*Gidlund* et al. 1978).

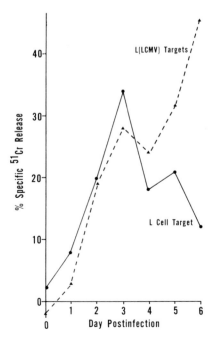

Fig. 1. Generation of cytotoxic spleen leukocytes from C3H/St mice infected with lymphocytic choriomeningitis virus (LCMV). Spleen leukocytes from 6-week-old mice infected intraperitoneally with $2 \times 10^4$ PFU of LCMV were tested for cytotoxicity against uninfected or LCMV-infected L-929 cells at effector to target ratios of 100:1 in a 16 h cytotoxicity assay. Reprinted with the permission of Nature (*Welsh* and *Zinkernagel* 1977)

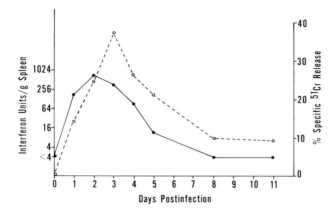

Fig. 2. Correlation of interferon levels and natural killer cell activity in spleens of LCMV-infected C3H/St mice. L-929 cells were used as targets in 16 h cytotoxicity assays. ●--●--● interferon; O--O--O cytotoxicity. Reprinted with the permission of The Journal of Experimental Medicine (*Welsh* 1978b)

The level of the NK cell response to a viral infection should depend on at least two major phenomena: 1. the ability of the virus to replicate in the host and induce interferon, and 2. the genetically determined levels of host NK activity. Different viruses vary in regard to their ability to induce NK cell activity in vivo (*Herberman* et al. 1977). This is probably a function of their ability to induce interferon production in NK-rich organs such as the spleen. Hence, lymphotropic viruses may be better NK cell activators than viruses with other types of selective organotropisms. Obviously, if a mouse is genetically resistant to a virus infection, the level of NK cell response may be low. Data showing a parallel between enhanced NK cell activity and recovery from a virus infection should be carefully scrutinized, since high interferon levels will accompany the high NK activity and interferon itself may inhibit virus synthesis (*Isaacs* and *Lindenmann* 1957). Alternatively, data showing an inverse relationship between enhanced NK activity and resistance to virus infection (*Gee* et al. 1980) should also be interpreted carefully, because the synthesis of more virus should result in the induction of more interferon and consequently greater NK cell activation.

Virus replication in the absence of an interferon response fails to induce NK-cell activity (*Hansson* et al. 1980). Adult mice persistently infected from birth with LCMV carry virus for life in the blood, spleen, and other major organs (*Traub* 1936), but they have levels of NK cell activity comparable to control mice (*Hansson* et al., 1980) and no detectable interferon levels (*Volkert* et al. 1964; *Hansson* et al. 1980). The titers of infectious LCMV in these persistently infected mice are, however, significantly lower than those in acutely infected mice, and this may account for the reduced interferon response.

The question of interferon induction in vivo by LCMV is rather complicated because the virus is a very poor interferon inducer in vitro (*Welsh* and *Pfau* 1972). It is not known if interferon produced in vivo is synthesized by only certain types of specialized cells in response to the LCMV infection. Since interferon is produced within hours of infection of normal and athymic nude mice, and is of the type I variety (*Merigan* et al. 1977; *Reviere* et al. 1977; *Bro-Jorgensen* 1978; *Welsh* 1978b), it does in this circumstance seem to be produced as a direct consequence of virus infection and not as a consequence of the immune response. However, viruses may also induce interferon production by lymphoid cells immunologically responding to infection. Hence, different types of interferon synthesized by different cells during the course of the viral infection may contribute to the activation of the NK cell. We have examined this in the LCMV system and found that the shape of the cytotoxicity curve shown in Figure 1 changes with the duration of the cytotoxicity assay because of apparent in vitro activation of NK cells (*Welsh* and *Doe*, 1980). Figure 3 shows that if spleen cells from LCMV-infected mice are cultured overnight before use as effectors, the only nonspecific NK cell-like cytotoxicity that can be detected occurs during the advent of the virus-specific cytotoxic T-cell response. Mouse NK-cell activity is unstable in culture, but in this system the NK activity 6 days postinfection appears to be stabilized by high levels of acid-labile (type II) interferon produced in the culture. Depletion of T cells from the culture with an antibody to Thy 1.2 antigen plus complement completely eliminates the interferon production (*Welsh* and *Doe*, 1980). Thus, assays for NK cells probably reflect both their levels of activity in vivo and their ability to be activated by immunologically responding cells in vitro. Such immune interferon associated with virus-specific cytotoxic T cells might also serve to activate NK cells in local areas of specific immunologic attack.

Activation of NK cells by a secondary challenge in immune mice is inhibited. Infection of control mice with $2 \times 10^4$ (low dose) or $2 \times 10^7$ (high dose) of LCMV plaque-forming units (PFU) leads to an activated NK cell response. However, only the high dose induces NK cell activity in LCMV-immune mice (*Biron* and *Welsh*, unpublished work).

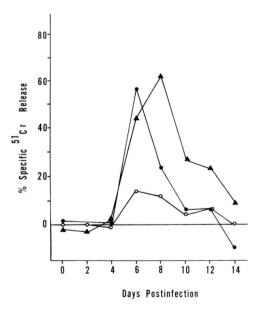

Fig. 3. Cytotoxicity by overnight-cultured leukocytes from LCMV-infected C3H/St mice. Spleen leukocytes from mice different days post infection were cultured for 16 h at 37 °C and then exposed to targets in a 16 h cytotoxicity assay. Targets: O-O-O, L-929 cells; ●-●-●, F-9 cells; ▲-▲-▲, LCMV-infected L-929 cells. For further details, see *Welsh* and *Doe* (1980)

A low dose of LCMV does elicit activated NK cells in Pichinde virus (PV)-immune mice, and a low dose of PV activates NK cells in LCMV-immune but not PV-immune mice (*Welsh* 1978b). The reason for this appears to be simply a function of interferon levels, as interferon production is very low in LCMV immune mice challenged with LCMV (*Biron, Kunkel* and *Welsh*, unpublished work). Presumably, the rapid induction of the memory-immune response curtails the spread of virus and the resulting interferon synthesis, as suggested in other systems (*Baron* 1970).

LCMV induces NK cell activity in all tested strains of mice, including both high and low NK reactive strains (*Welsh* 1978b), nude mice (*Herberman* et al. 1977; *Welsh* and *Zinkernagel* 1977), and NK-deficient beige mice (*Welsh* and *Kiessling* 1980; *Talmadge* et al. 1980a, b). The augmentation of NK-cell activity by LCMV generally parallels at a higher level the uninduced endogenous NK activity in regard to strain distribution and age of mice (*Welsh* 1978b; *Kiessling* and *Welsh* 1980; *Welsh* and *Kiessling* 1980). NK activity can also be augmented by LCMV infection of newborn mice (*Welsh* 1978b), which at one time were reported to have virtually no endogenous NK cell activity (*Kiessling* et al. 1975a; *Herberman* et al. 1975). Sex does not influence the levels of endogenous NK cells nor does it seem to affect the in vivo activation of NK cells by LCMV (*Welsh* 1978b). However, female but not male BALB/C mice develop NK cell-like activity in response to Coxsackie B-3 virus infection (*Wong* et al. 1977). The reason for the sex difference in the Coxsackie infection is not understood, but sex differences were also reported in regards to the cytotoxic T cell response.

Activated NK cells can be induced by virus infections in X-ray-irradiated mice, indicating that cell division is not required for activation, but the levels of induced NK activity are significantly lower than in unirradiated mice (*Welsh* 1978b). Virus-induced NK cell activity is also reduced after bone marrow irradiation with [89]Sr (*Welsh* 1978b), while athymic nude mice respond to viral infections with rather high levels of NK activity (*Herberman* et al. 1977; *Welsh* and *Zinkernagel* 1977; *Welsh* 1978b).

## 2.3 Factors Regulating the Decline of NK Activity

The mechanisms behind the decline of the enhanced NK cell activity in virus-infected animals (Fig. 1) have not been defined but can probably be logically deduced. A fall in NK activity usually parallels a fall in the level of interferon (*Welsh* 1978b; Fig 2). Since interferon is induced directly by the virus infection or indirectly by the immune response to the virus infection, the presence of the virus or viral antigens would in either case be required for continued interferon production. Thus, factors contributing to the clearance of the virus, such as viral interference phenomena or specific immune response mechanisms, should consequently reduce the interferon levels required for NK cell activation. NK cell activity in LCMV-infected nude mice, which do not clear the infection, remains elevated long after NK cell levels have declined in nude/+ controls (*Welsh* 1978b), suggesting that the T-cell-dependent immune response, known to clear the LCMV infection in vivo (*Zinkernagel* and *Welsh* 1976), ultimately contributes to the shutdown of interferon synthesis and activated NK cells.

Other mechanisms may exist for a more direct shutdown of NK cell activity during virus infections. Cells which suppress NK activity have been found in mice infected with *Corynebacterium parvum* (*Savary* and *Lotzova* 1978) or Bacille-Calmette-Guerin (BCG)

(*Ito* et al. 1980). Such suppressor cells may also appear during virus infections. LCMV infection also leads to a marked degeneration of the bone marrow, accompanied by a significant reduction in pluripotential stem cells (colony-forming units) developing from such marrow (*Bro-Jorgensen* 1978). Since NK cell precursors may be bone marrow derived (*Haller* and *Wigzell* 1977; *Haller* et al. 1977), it seems possible that a depletion in the generation of NK cells could occur at some time during a virus infection. Interestingly, this bone marrow depletion may be a direct effect of interferon (*Bro-Jorgensen* 1978). Hence, the same factor that activates NK cells could potentially also contribute to a reduction in NK cell number or activity. Research in this area should be pursued.

## 2.4 Characteristics of NK Cells Activated in Vivo

Natural killer cells activated during the LCMV infection share most of the characteristics of endogenous cells, with a few quantitative exceptions. The virus-activated cells are more adherent to nylon wool, plastic surfaces, and antibody-coated erythrocyte (EA) monolayers (*Kiessling* et al. 1980). Adherence to EA monolayers can be prevented by IgG Fc-binding staphylococcal A protein, suggesting that activated NK cells bind via Fc receptors. Those activated NK cells which pass through nylon wool columns do not express these higher levels of Fc receptors, suggesting that the nylon wool adherent and high Fc receptor containing cells may represent similar or overlapping cell populations (*Kiessling* et al. 1980). LCMV-activated NK cells in some instances have enhanced sensitivity to lysis with antibody to Thy 1.2 and complement (*Herberman* et al. 1978; *Kiessling* et al. 1980), and two reports suggest that large blast-size cells contain NK cell activity after virus infection (*Tai* et al. 1980; *Kiessling* et al. 1980). It is not known, however, whether NK cells undergo blastogenesis during the course of a viral infection.

## 2.5 Induction of NK Cell Activity by Virus Infections in Man

Little is known about the induction of NK cell activity in man by acute virus infections. Most studies of this nature have been unsuccessful searches for HLA-restricted virus specific T cells or fruitful studies on K cell-mediated ADCC, which rises in parallel with the production of antiviral antibody in vivo and in culture (*Perrin* et al. 1977; *Greenberg* et al. 1980). Undoubtedly, information on NK cell activation in man will soon be forthcoming. This can be predicted because virus infections induce interferon production in man (*Wheelock* and *Sibley* 1964), and administration of interferon to human cancer patients has resulted in elevated levels of NK cell activity in human peripheral blood leukocytes (PBL) (*Huddlestone* et al. 1979; *Einhorn* et al. 1978). For the reasons discussed in Sect. 2.2, it can be predicted that activated NK cells will be found during acute virus infections of humans but probably not in subjects receiving secondary immunizations. Such individuals could well develop an anamnestic antibody response correlating with enhanced K cell activity in the absence of elevated NK cell activity.

# 3 Induction of NK Cell Activity by Virus Infection in Vitro

## 3.1 Human Studies

While the mouse has provided the bulk of knowledge concerning NK cell activation in vivo, the in vitro induction of NK cell activity was first documented and most elegantly described using human PBL. Virus-infected fibroblasts exposed to human PBL are usually lysed at higher levels than uninfected fibroblasts (Table 2). *Santoli* et al. (1978a, b) showed that this superficially "specific" killing of virus infected targets was actually due to the activation of NK cells in the virus-infected cultures. Virus-infected cells or virus alone induced the synthesis of interferon in the PBL. The production of interferon paralleled the induction of NK cell activity (*Santoli* et al. 1978b), and the interferon was shown to be of sufficient quantities to activate NK cells (*Santoli* et al. 1978b; *Trinchieri* and *Santoli* 1978). Using a number of viruses (e.g., influenza, HSV-1, paramyxoviruses) these investigators showed that the lysis of targets was best achieved during a 16 h incubation, as opposed to a shorter cytotoxicity assay. This allowed sufficient time for interferon synthesis and subsequent NK cell activation. The interferon produced in the influenza cytotoxicity assays was greater than 10 000 units/0.1 ml, far in excess of levels required to activate NK cells (*Santoli* et al. 1978b).

## 3.2 Mouse Studies

Essentially similar findings to the above have been found in the mouse system, where lysis of acutely infected (*Anderson* 1978; *Welsh* and *Hallenback* 1980) or persistently infected (*Minato* et al. 1979) cultures by endogenous spleen cells is higher than that of uninfected cultures. This lysis is associated with interferon synthesis, requires an overnight incubation to develop, and results in a generalized elevation of NK cell activity. One problem with the interpretation of these studies is that the production of interferon is

Table 2. Lysis of virus-infected cells after incubation with normal leukocytes in vitro

| Virus | Effector cell | References |
|---|---|---|
| Cytomegalo | Human | *Diamond* et al. 1977 |
| Epstein-Barr | Human | *Blazar* et al. 1980 |
| HSV-1 | Human | *Santoli* et al. 1978a; *Ching* and *Lopez* 1979 |
| HSV-1 | Mouse | *Welsh* and *Hallenbeck* 1980 |
| Influenza | Human | *Santoli* et al. 1978a, b |
| Measles | Human | *Santoli* et al. 1978a; *Ault* and *Weiner* 1979 |
| Measles | Mouse | *Minato* et al. 1979 |
| Mumps | Human | *Harfast* et al. 1978; *Santoli* and *Trinchieri* 1978a |
| Mumps | Mouse | *Minato* et al. 1979 |
| Paramyxo | Human | *Santoli* et al. 1978a |
| Sendai | Mouse | *Anderson* 1978; *Welsh* and *Hallenbeck* 1980 |
| Sindbis | Mouse | *Welsh* and *Hallenbeck* 1980 |
| Vesicular stomatitis | Mouse | *Minato* et al. 1979; *Welsh* and *Hallenbeck* 1980 |

much lower (< 500 U/ml) than that in the human system (*Reid* et al., to be published; *Welsh* and *Hallenbeck* 1980), and we have not been able to activate NK cells in vitro by the direct addition of these tissue culture supernatants. Perhaps the incubation of NK cells in proximity to interferon-producing cells or else the production of interferon by the mouse NK cells themselves may lead to more efficient activation.

## 3.3 Non-Interferon-Associated Mechanisms?

While it is clear that viruses induce interferon and that interferon activates NK cells, it is not clear that this represents the only mechanism for enhanced natural killing. Perhaps the most extensively studied system in this regard is that of mumps virus. Mumps virus-infected cells are lysed at high efficiency by human PBL with the characteristics of NK cells (*Andersson* et al. 1975; *Harfast* et al. 1975; *Harfast* et al. 1978). Fab (antigen-binding fragments) directed against human IgG failed to prevent the lysis, indicating that the cytotoxicity was not mediated by antibody (*Harfast* et al. 1978). What is interesting in this system is that PBL pretreated with mumps virus alone, UV-inactivated mumps virus, or mumps virus glycoprotein also exhibited enhanced cytotoxicity against a panel of unin-fected target cells in 16 h cytotoxicity assays. Although initially identified as classical NK cells (*Harfast* et al. 1980a), the effector cells in this system have recently been shown to be heterogeneous in regards to expressing Fc receptors, i.e., some do not express any detec-table Fc receptors (*A. Alsheikhly*, unpublished work). While not ruling out an interferon-mediated activation, *Harfast* et al. (1980b) could detect no interferon production under these assay conditions.

   A similar study in our laboratory has produced some comparable results with measles virus (*Casali, Sissons* and *Oldstone*, unpublished work). Infection of human PBL with measles virus for 16 h results in the production of interferon and development of NK cytotoxicity similar to that reported by *Santoli* et al. (1978a, b). However, if PBL and unin-fected target cells (human fibroblasts) are mixed with measles virus glycoprotein, either alone or incorporated into liposomes, there is a rapid onset of cytotoxicity (within 4 h) in the absence of detectable interferon synthesis. The mechanism of this apparent rapid activation is not known, though one could speculate that the binding of the glycoprotein to the effector cell may function as an analogue of interferon (which also is a cell surface binding glycoprotein) and induce an effect in the cell similar to that induced by inter-feron. Alternatively, viral glycoproteins may possibly enhance lysis by agglutinating or fusing effector cells to target cells. In several virus infections, a rapid enhanced lysis of virus-infected targets in association with enhanced binding of effectors to the target cells has been reported. These include various cell types infected with measles virus (*Ault* and *Weiner* 1979), Epstein-Barr virus (EBV) (*Blazer* et al. 1980), Sendai virus (*Welsh* and *Hallenbeck* 1980), and mouse hepatitis virus (MHV) (*Holmes, Haspel* and *Welsh*, un-published work). Because of the short assay times, it is difficult to ascribe a classical inter-feron-dependent mechanism to these systems. The subject of NK cell recognition of virus-infected targets is discussed in Sect. 4.

## 3.4 NK Cell Activation Associated with Immune Response in Vitro

NK-like cytotoxicity can be demonstrated under conditions of lymphocyte stimulation in vitro. In addition to the cytotoxic T cells with specificity for alloantigens, mixed lymphocyte cultures induce effector cells with broad specificities similar to NK cells (*Seeley* and *Golub* 1978; *Karre* and *Seeley* 1979; *Zarling* and *Bach* 1978). Such NK-like cytotoxic cells are also generated in response to allogeneic and autologous EBV cell lines (*Svedmyr* and *Jondal* 1975; *Svedmyr* et al. 1974; *Jondal* and *Targan* 1978; *Biron* et al. 1981). It is not clear at this time whether these cells are true NK cells. The in vitro induced effector cells differ from freshly isolated NK cells in that there is reduced expression of Fc receptors (*Jondal* and *Targan* 1978; *Seeley* et al. 1979) and enhanced levels of cytotoxicity associated with blast-size cells (*Karre* and *Seeley* 1979; *Biron* et al. 1981). Similar types of cytotoxic cells can also be generated during secondary stimulation with UV-inactivated EB virions (*Hutt-Fletcher* and *Gilbert*, to be published). The potential role of NK cells in EB viral infections will be discussed in Sect. 5.4.

## 4 Virus-Induced Alteration of Target Cell Susceptibility to NK-Cell-Mediated Lysis

To define the role of NK cells in virus infections, one must not only consider the ability of viruses to induce NK cell activity but also the ability of viruses to affect the susceptibility of target cells. The original studies on target specificities of mouse NK cells led to the hypothesis that NK cells recognized RNA tumor virus (retrovirus) antigens on the target cell surface (*Herberman* et al. 1975; *Kiessling* et al. 1975a). Lymphoma cells expressing these antigens appeared more sensitive than other cells to natural killing. It was suggested that the 3- to 4-week duration after birth before NK cells could be detected provided time for the NK cells to respond immunologically against retrovirus antigens and develop cytotoxicity against target cells expressing those antigens (*Herberman* et al. 1975). This implied that the internal viral environment of the mouse influenced endogenous NK cell activity. However, cell transfer experiments showed that the development of NK cell activity was exclusively a function of the bone marrow and not of the genetic and viral background of the host (*Haller* et al. 1977). More extensive studies with endogenous NK cells failed to show a preferential killing of retroviral antigen-expressing cells (*Becker* and *Klein* 1976; *Becker* et al. 1976), and superinfection of human cell lines with a xenotropic murine retrovirus did not confer an enhanced sensitivity to these targets (*Kiessling* et al. 1978). Activated mouse NK cells were shown to lyse xenogeneic (human) cells not expressing detectable retroviral antigens and to lyse normal and tumor mouse cells whether or not they expressed such antigens (*Nunn* et al. 1977; *Welsh* and *Zinkernagel* 1977; *Welsh* et al. 1979; *MacFarlan* et al. 1979). It can be concluded that the expression of retroviral antigens is not required for natural killing, though some role of these antigens in the interaction between target and effector cells cannot be ruled out.

The duration of this discussion will consider the effects of viruses other than retroviruses on the sensitivity of target cells. While many studies have reported that such virus-infected cells are more sensitive than uninfected cells to NK cell mediated lysis, only recently have investigators taken into account the fact that viruses can activate NK cells in vitro to kill nonspecifically. Most of the interpretable data on target cell sensitivities can only be derived from short-term assays where additional NK cell activation is minimal. Even under those conditions, some type of interferon-dependent activation mechanism is difficult to rule out. Results to date have indicated that viral infections may either enhance, inhibit, or not change the susceptibility of target cells to NK-cell-mediated lysis.

## 4.1 Interferon-Induced Resistance of Target Cells to NK Cell-Mediated Lysis

*Trinchieri* and *Santoli* (1978) reported that interferon treatment could render normal human target cells resistant to NK-cell-mediated lysis. Subsequent work has shown that both human and mouse normal and tumor target cells are protected by species-specific interferon (*Moore* et al. 1980; *Welsh* et al. 1981). These interferon-treated targets are susceptible to ADCC and cytotoxic T cell killing. Interferon-treated targets fail to inhibit NK cell mediated lysis in cold target competition assays (*Trinchieri* and *Santoli* 1978; *Welsh* et al. 1981), suggesting that the nature of the binding of the NK cell to the target cell is affected. The biochemical basis of this protection is not understood, but recent work from our group has indicated that interferon causes an increase in glycolipid-associated cell surface sialic acid on several cell lines and that at least in some circumstances the presence of high concentrations of cell surface sialic acid correlates with resistance to NK cells (*Yogeeswaran, Gronberg, Hansson, Kiessling, Fujinami* and *Welsh*, unpublished works).

Infection of human fibroblasts with either of several viruses rendered them resistant to the interferon-mediated protection (*Trinchieri* and *Santoli* 1978). This presumably was due to the fact that viruses commonly inhibit cellular RNA and protein synthesis whose induction is required for interferon-mediated effects. On the basis of those results, *Trinchieri* and *Santoli* (1978) proposed that during a virus infection the virus-induced interferon will activate NK cells and protect uninfected target cells, but will leave virus-infected target cells sensitive to NK cell mediated lysis. In this way, NK cells could function to selectively eliminate virus-infected cells and therefore play a major role in nonspecific resistance to virus infections. This hypothesis is both appealing and reasonable. However, it should only apply to certain viruses and in certain types of virus-infected cells, since many viruses are noncytopathic or else do not significantly inhibit host RNA and protein synthesis until very late in the infection. Further work in this regard would be of interest.

## 4.2 Reduced Sensitivity of Virus-Infected Target Cells to NK Cell-Mediated Lysis

We have examined the sensitivities of virus-infected L-929 cells to activated NK cells in short-term assays and have found that virus-infected cells (e.g., by Sendai virus, vesicular stomatitis virus, Sindbis virus, HSV) commonly become more resistant to lysis (*Welsh* and *Hallenbeck* 1980). Interferon is produced in these virus-infected cultures, but whether interferon mediates this protection is not known. Interestingly, Sendai virus-infected L-929 cells express the viral hemagglutinin and bind to lymphocytes with some selectivity for NK cells. Though resistant to NK cell-mediated lysis, the Sendai virus infected L-929 cells are, however, sensitive to anti-H-2$^k$ ADCC. Thus, resistance to NK may be conferred by a virus infection, and such resistance may be due to factors other than simple binding of the effector to the target cell (*Welsh* and *Hallenbeck* 1980).

Vero cells infected with HSV-1 become very resistant to NK cell-mediated lysis, and this virus-induced resistance cannot be explained by interferon, since vero cells do not produce it (*Welsh* and *Hallenbeck* 1980). As shown by direct-target cell binding or indirectly by cold-target competition assays, HSV-infected vero cells did not bind to NK cells and therefore resisted lysis. The specific biochemical mechanism for this is not known, though HSV infection causes alterations in cell surface glycoproteins and glycolipids (*Schroder* and *Merrick* 1979).

## 4.3 Increased Sensitivity of Virus-Infected Target Cells to NK Cell-Mediated Lysis

In most studies using activated NK cells in short-term assays, virus-infected target cells do not have enhanced sensitivity to NK cell-mediated lysis (*Santoli* et al. 1978a, b; *Trinchieri* and *Santoli* 1978; *Welsh* and *Hallenbeck* 1980). However, this is not always the case, as Sendai virus-infected vero cells have heightened sensitivity to activated mouse NK cells in assays as short as 1 h (*Welsh* and *Hallenbeck* 1980). These targets bound effectors more efficiently than uninfected cells.

Enhanced binding of endogenous NK cells concomitant with enhanced lysis of virus-infected targets in short-term assays has been reported in several systems, including measles virus (*Ault* and *Weiner* 1979), EBV (*Blazar* et al. 1979), and Sendai virus (*Welsh* and *Hallenbeck* 1980). Whether NK cell activation occurs under these conditions is not well understood (see Sect. 3.2). An additional point to be considered in this regard is the influence of the target cell. Whereas Sendai virus-infected vero cells have enhanced sensitivity to endogenous or activated NK cells, Sendai-virus-infected L-929 cells are markedly resistant to lysis by activated effectors (*Welsh* and *Hallenbeck* 1980).

## 4.4 Virus-Elicited Factors Which Could Influence the Sensitivity of Target Cells to NK Cell-Mediated Lysis

Viral infections have the capability to influence target cell susceptibility to NK cells by known as well as potential mechanisms. These include the following:
1. Interferon-mediated protection, as discussed in Sect. 4.1.
2. Enhanced binding or fusion to effectors via hemagglutinin- and hemolysin(fusion)-type virus-coded cell surface glycoproteins, as discussed in Sect. 4.3. The possibility also exists that viruses could induce increased expression of the target moiety recognized by NK cells on the cytoplasmic membrane.
3. Direct protection of target cells by biochemical alterations in the cell membrane preventing NK cell binding and/or lysis, as discussed in Sect. 4.2.
4. Enhanced sensitivity of target cells due to virus-induced inhibition of membrane repair. This potential mechanism for selective lysis of virus-infected cells has thus far not been described. However, we have found that actinomycin D, an inhibitor of RNA synthesis, and cycloheximide, an inhibitor of protein synthesis, confer an enhanced sensitivity of L-929 cells to NK cell-mediated lysis (*Kunkel* and *Welsh*, Int. J. Cancer, in press). Similar treatments have been shown to enhance target cell sensitivity to complement-mediated lysis and have been correlated with defects in membrane repair (*Schlager* et al. 1977, 1978; *Schreiber* et al. 1980). Since many virus infections can inhibit cellular RNA and protein synthesis, such a mechanism should be considered for the enhanced sensitivity of virus-infected targets to NK cells.

## 4.5 Specificity and Restriction in Lysing Virus-Infected Cells

Most reports claiming specific recognition of virus-infected targets by NK cells can now be dismissed in view of current evidence concerning NK cell activation. However, *Minato* et al. (1979), using BHK and Hela cells persistently infected with a variety of viruses [measles, influenza, mumps, vesicular stomatitis virus (VSV), etc.] reported that the lysis of Hela cells persistently infected with measles virus could be inhibited by homologous cells in cold-target competition assays but not by uninfected or VSV-infected Hela cells or by uninfected or virus-infected baby hamster kidney (BHK) cells. This result conflicts with most other reports on NK cells and requires further study and confirmation.

   *Anderson* (1978) reported that NK cell-mediated lysis of Sendai virus-infected L-929 cells was H-2 restricted. Unfortunately, only one target was used, and the effectors which were H-2 compatible with the target were from highly NK reactive strains (*Petranyi* et al. 1976), while those which were incompatible and failed to lyse the target were from low NK strains. We have not seen H-2 restriction in the lysis of Sendai virus-infected L-929 cells (*Welsh* and *Hallenbeck* 1980), and virtually all reports with other viruses have failed to demonstrate H-2 specific NK cell killing. The conclusions of Anderson's paper concerning H-2 restriction can therefore probably be disregarded.

## 5 Role of NK Cells During Virus Infection in Vivo

At the time of this writing there is no firm evidence that NK cells play a role in virus infection in vivo. Athymic nude mice are particularly susceptible to virus infections, even though high levels of NK activity are induced in such infections (*Herberman* et al. 1977; *Welsh* and *Zinkernagel* 1977; *Welsh* 1978b). In the only experiments thus far published using NK cell-deficient (*Roder* and *Duwe* 1979) beige mice, no differences in the production of LCMV PFU's were seen early in the infection (*Welsh* and *Kiessling* 1980). However, some promising data have come from mouse genetic studies which link susceptibility to virus infection with the hemopoietic histocompatibility (Hh) system (*Cudkowicz* and *Lotzova* 1973). The Hh system refers to the genetically determined ability of mice to reject certain grafts of normal and neoplastic hemopoietic cells, notably in $F_1$ hybrid recipients of parental bone marrow (*Cudkowicz* and *Bennett* 1971). There are marked similarities between the effector cells of the Hh system and NK cells, including:

1. Maturation during the 4th week of life; 2. Low sensitivity to whole-body X-ray-irradiation; 3. Maturation independent of the thymus; 4. Dependence on the integrity of the bone marrow; 5. Suppression by injections of antimacrophage agents (silica and carrageenan); and 6. Suppression by multiple injections of parental spleen cells into $F_1$ mice (*Kiessling* et al. 1977). From the above data it would appear that the Hh graft rejection is mediated by an NK cell or a cell similar to it.

### 5.1 Resistance to Friend Virus

Substantial work by *Kumar, Bennett*, and co-workers has indicated that the resistance of mice to the Friend virus (FV) complex may be mediated by an NK-like cell (*Kumar* et al. 1974, 1976, 1978; *Kumar* and *Bennett* 1976). The FV complex consists of spleen focus-forming virus (SFFV) and lymphatic leukemia virus (LLV) and causes both a progressing erythroleukemia and profound immunosuppression in mice. Susceptibility to both the erythropoietic and immunosuppressive effects is controlled by several genes, but mice which are particularly resistant to bone marrow allografts tend to resist the FV infection (*Kumar* et al. 1974). Resistance to FV can be transferred with bone marrow (*Axelrad* and *Van Der Gaag* 1968; *Odaka* and *Matsukura* 1969), but aborted by treatment of mice with the bone marrow-seeking isotope $^{89}$Sr (*Kumar* et al. 1974). Further delineation of the system in vitro showed that a bone-marrow-derived cell, called an "M" cell by these investigators, appeared to regulate the functions of T suppressor cells, which mediated the FV-induced immunosuppression (*Kumar* and *Bennett* 1976; *Kumar* et al. 1976).

## 5.2 Resistance to Herpesvirus

Correlations between the Hh system and resistance to HSV-1 infection have also been made (*Lopez* 1975, 1978; *Lopez* and *Bennett* 1978). In addition to strain-dependent similarities between resistance to HSV and resistance to bone marrow allografts, direct studies using bone marrow transfers and $^{89}$Sr indicated a function for bone marrow in resistance (*Lopez* and *Bennett* 1978). Treatment of resistant mice with $^{89}$Sr resulted in a spread of virus to the spinal cord, suggesting that "M" cells may inhibit the spread of virus. HSV-infected targets are good inducers of mouse and human NK activity in vitro (*Santoli* et al. 1978a; *Ching* and *Lopez* 1979; *Welsh* and *Hallenbeck* 1980). While there is some preliminary indication that NK activity may be elevated during normal human HSV infections, two tested humans suffering from severe disseminated Herpesvirus infections had low NK activity (*Ching* and *Lopez* 1979).

## 5.3 Resistance to Mouse Hepatitis Virus

Resistance of mice to infection with MHV is age dependent and can be conferred by transfer of cells from adult mice into newborns (*Levy-LeBlond* and *Dupuy* 1978). Such experiments indicated that three cell populations were required for transfer of resistance: adherent spleen cells, T cells, and bone marrow cells. The bone marrow cells required in the transfer had many properties in common with NK cells, including organ distribution (present in bone marrow, spleen, and peritoneum and absent in thymus), age of maturation, lability in culture, nonadherence to plastic, sensitivity to $^{89}$Sr, and enhancement by BCG (*Tardieu* et al. 1980). In our hands, MHV-infected targets are acutely sensitive to lysis by normal mouse leukocytes in short-term assays ($< 4$ h), suggesting a possible direct effector function of NK-like cells in this system (*Holmes, Haspel* and *Welsh*, unpublished work).

## 5.4 Resistance to Epstein-Barr Virus

The role of NK cells in EBV infection in man has been the subject of much research but remains speculative. It is unclear whether EBV infection induces NK cell activity. PBL isolated from individuals with infectious mononucleosis demonstrate spontaneous killing (*Svedmyr* and *Jondal* 1975; *Hutt* et al. 1975; *Bakacs* et al. 1978). This activity was originally reported as separating with either the null cell or Fc-receptor positive T cell population (*Bakacs* et al. 1978). Normal PBL can inhibit the outgrowth of newly infected B cells (*Thorley-Lawson* et al. 1977), and the effector cell in this system was reported to be a T lymphocyte with Fc receptors for IgG (*Shope* and *Kaplan* 1979). The distinction between these T cells with IgG Fc receptors and NK cells is unclear, since they might belong to the same cell population. Although EBV-carrying cell lines are not always lysed by NK cells (*Jondal* et al. 1978), a distinctly increased sensitivity to NK can be demonstrated when such cells are induced to express the late viral antigens which appear in productive infections (*Blazar* et al. 1980). Patients with X-linked lymphoproliferative syndrome have a genetic deficiency which renders them particularly sensitive to EBV infection, commonly resulting in lymphoma (*Purtillo* et al. 1977). These patients have recently been shown to have reduced levels of NK cells in their peripheral blood (*Sullivan* et al. 1980).

# 6 NK Cells as Producers of Interferon

In addition to being activated by interferon, NK cells may produce interferon. Human cell populations enriched for NK cells produce high levels of interferon when exposed to viruses or tumor cells (*Trinchieri* et al. 1978), and antibody to leukocyte type 1 interferon binds to NK-enriched lymphocytes which bind to K562 cells (*E. Saxsela*, personal communication). Treatment of mouse spleen cells with antibody and complement to Ly 5, known to somewhat selectively lyse NK cells (*Young* et al. 1980; *Glimcher* et al. 1977), abrogates virus-induced interferon production (*Reid* et al., to be published). Therefore, in addition to their cytolytic capacities, NK cells may play an important role in virus infection by secreting interferon, which can directly inhibit virus synthesis.

# 7 Effect of Virus Infections on Tumorigenesis

Oncogenic viruses have the capacity to transform normal cells, rendering them capable of forming tumors in vivo. NK cells have been strongly implicated as factors inhibiting the development of such tumors induced by retroviruses in mice (reviewed by *Kiessling* and *Wigzell* 1979; *Kasai* et al. 1979) and by Marek's disease virus in chickens (*Lam* and *Linna* 1979). However, it has been known for years that certain acute virus infections may actually inhibit tumor growth (*Molomut* and *Padnos* 1965; *Yamada* and *Hatano* 1972). This has not been surprising, since viruses induce interferon and interferon can directly inhibit tumor cell division (*Gresser* et al. 1974). However, interferon treatment of mice implanted with an interferon-resistant tumor resulted in the rejection of the tumor (*Gresser* et al. 1972). This led Gresser and his colleagues to propose that interferon may function to inhibit tumor growth by inducing a host response mechanism.

The virus-induced resistance of mice to tumors has recently been studied in nude mice, which have high NK activity but poor specific immune response mechanisms. *Kuzumaki* and *Koboyashi* (1976) first showed that nude mice implanted with retrovirus- or paramyxovirus-infected tumor cells either did not form tumors or had reduced tumor growth. This indicated that T cells and T cell-dependent functions were not responsible for the tumor rejection. *Reid* et al. (1979) further investigated this system, showing that xenogeneic BHK or Hela cells persistently infected with any of a number of RNA viruses (measles, influenza, mumps, rabies, vesicular stomatitis) either failed to form tumors or formed only small nodules in nude mice. Virus-infected tumor cells implanted in X-ray-irradiated mice did form tumors, again suggesting that a host response was responsible for the inhibition of tumor cell growth (*Kuzumaki* and *Koboyashi* 1976; *Reid* et al. 1979). Additional studies in the system produced the expected results showing that the virus-infected tumor cells induced interferon and NK cell activity in vivo and in vitro when exposed to mouse spleen cells (*Minato* et al. 1979; *Reid* et al., to be published). Mice treated with antilymphocyte serum or with antibody to mouse interferon developed tumors when implanted with virus-infected cells (*Reid* et al., to be published). All these data are consistent with the hypothesis that virus-induced interferon-activated NK cells inhibited the growth of virus-infected tumors. Nevertheless, the results are not conclusive, as other effector cells such as macrophages are not ruled out by these experiments. It does seem clear that the tumor rejection required interferon synthesis, but recent work by Blalock and colleagues suggests that a direct interferon-mediated inhibition of tumor growth cannot be ignored, even when xenogeneic tumor cells are used. These investigators have shown that interferon induces an antiviral activity which can be transferred directly to cells lacking receptors for that species of interferon if the cells are in contact with each other (*Blalock* et al. 1979). The ability of interferon to actually protect tumor cells from NK cell-mediated lysis (*Moore* et al. 1980; *Welsh* et al. 1981) also casts some questions on whether the tumor rejections are NK cell mediated. However, if NK cells are the major producers of interferon in response to tumors or virus infections, as discussed in Sect. 6, they may be functionally important by mechanisms additional to their cytolytic capabilities.

Further evidence that NK cells may be directly involved in the rejection of virus-infected tumor cells comes from experiments with NK cell-deficient beige (bg) mice. C57BL/6 bg/bg mice have low cytotoxic NK cell levels (*Roder* and *Duwe* 1979) which can be augmented by LCMV infection (*Welsh* and *Kiessling* 1980; *Talmadge* et al. 1980a, b). Interferon synthesis in LCMV-infected beige mice is comparable to that of infected normal mice (*Welsh* and *Kiessling* 1980). In a series of elegant experiments, Talmadge and co-workers have shown bg/bg but not bg/+ mice to be highly sensitive to tumor formation and metastases by an NK-sensitive tumor cell implant. After infection with LCMV, the beige mice became resistant to tumor formation by these cells and developed NK cytotoxic activity against them. Under these same conditions, cells selected to be NK resistant were not rejected by the bg/bg mice. In short-term assays measuring the clearance of IUDR-labeled tumor cells in bg/bg and bg/+ mice, *Talmadge* et al. (1980b) demonstrated a marked enhancement in the clearing of NK sensitive cells in vivo, if mice were first infected with LCMV. We find that fibroblasts infected with LCMV and radiolabeled with $^{125}$IUDR are cleared more rapidly than uninfected cells from inoculated mice (*Biron* and *Welsh*, unpublished work). These experiments together imply a direct cytotoxic mechanism, since a tumor-growth-inhibiting effect by interferon should not influence retention of the label in so short a time period.

As discussed earlier, virus infections may influence the susceptibility of target cells to NK cell-mediated lysis. Since these infections commonly render cells more resistant to lysis (*Welsh* and *Hallenbeck* 1980; *Reid* et al., to be published), one could speculate that a persistent virus infection may actually increase the tumorigenicity of cells. It is of course well known that many types of viruses transform cells, but here we are only considering the possibility of a virus-induced membrane alteration which renders a cell resistant to

NK cell-mediated surveillance. Such a situation has now been described (*Reid* et al., to be published; *Jones* et al. 1980). A BHK cell line persistently infected with VSV formed tumors in nude mice instead of being rejected like other virus-infected cells. Virus from these cells was used to infect other BHK cells. These newly infected cells formed tumors in mice and had decreased sensitivity to NK cell-mediated lysis. Nevertheless, these virus-infected cells induced interferon synthesis and NK cell activity in vivo and in vitro. These results suggest that the double event of cell transformation plus persistent virus infection could synergistically provide mechanisms for tumor development and metastasis.

## 8 K Cell-Mediated Lysis in Virus Infections

Antiviral ADCC can be mediated by polymorphonuclear leukocytes (*Grewal* et al. 1977), macrophages (*MacFarlan* et al. 1977), and lymphocytes. The most commonly reported effector of antiviral ADCC is a K lymphocyte with properties identical to or nearly identical to NK cells (see Sect. 1). K cell-mediated lysis has been documented with a number of human viruses, including HSV-1, mumps, measles, influenza, respiratory syncitial, and EB (reviewed by *Sissons* and *Oldstone*, to be published). K cell activity in PBL parallels the rise in antiviral antibody production following vaccination or acute infection (*Perrin* et al. 1978; *Meguro* et al. 1979; *Greenberg* et al. 1979, 1980). Discussion on the role of NK cells in virus infection must consider the potential ADCC capacity of such cells, and any data showing correlations between NK activity and virus disease may be a function of the specific rather than nonspecific manifestations of NK cells. See *Sissons* and *Oldstone* (to be published) for further discussions on this topic.

## 9 Summary and Conclusions

It is now apparent that NK cells are activated concomitantly with the induction of interferon synthesis during virus infections. These activated NK cells can lyse most normal and tumor target cells nonspecifically, but they may also serve as effector cells for specific antiviral ADCC. The role of NK cells in virus infections is unknown and difficult to predict, since cell culture studies indicate that virus-infected targets may become either more or less sensitive to natural killing. These targets all appear sensitive to ADCC, suggesting that if the nonspecific cytolytic capacity of the NK cell is ineffective, the antibody-mediated K cell function may be implemented. The strong possibility that NK cells are major interferon producers suggests that they may also play a role in resistance to virus infections by a mechanism other than cytotoxicity. There are some genetic data suggesting a role for NK-like cells in the resistance of mice to certain virus infections, and virus infections of tumor cells influence their tumorigenicity by mechanisms consistent with an NK cell-mediated hypothesis. Nevertheless, more sophisticated techniques which clearly distinguish NK cell mechanisms for other host defense mechanisms are required before conclusions can be made regarding the significance of the NK cells in virus infection in vivo.

*Acknowledgments.* This is publication No. 2200 from the Scripps Clinic and Research Foundation, La Jolla, California. This work was supported by U.S. Public Health Grants AI 12438, NS 12438, AI

07007, and Research Career Development Award AI 00253. I thank Drs. *Christine Biron* and *Bengt Harfast* for contributions to and critical review of the manuscript, Dr. *Michael Oldstone* for support, *Lori A. Kunkel* for technical assistance, and *Susan Edwards* for preparation of the manuscript.

# References

Anderson MJ (1978) Innate cytotoxicity of CBA mouse spleen cells to Sendai-virus infected L cells. Infect Immun 20:608–612

Andersson T, Steiskal V, Harfast B (1975) An in vitro method for study of human lymphocyte cytotoxicity against mumps virus-infected target cells. J Immunol 114:237–243

Ault KA, Weiner HL (1979) Natural killing of measles-infected cells by human lymphocytes. J Immunol 122:2616

Axelrad A, Gaag HC van der (1968) Genetic and cellular basis of susceptibility or resistance to Friend leukemia virus infection in mice. Proc Can Cancer Res Conf 8:313–343

Bakacs T Svedmyr E, Klein E, Rombo L, Weiland D (1978) EBV-related cytotoxicity of Fc receptor negative T lymphocytes separated from the blood of infectious mononucleosis patients. Cancer Lett 4:185–189

Baron S (1970) The defensive role of the interferon system. J Gen Physiol 56:193–211

Becker S, Klein E (1976) Decreased "Natural Killer" effect in tumor-bearing mice and its relation to the immunity against oncornavirus determined cell surface antigens. Eur J Immunol 6:892–898

Becker S, Fenyo EM, Klein E (1976) The "Natural Killer" cell in the mouse does not require H-2 homology and is not directed against type or group-specific antigens of murine C viral proteins. Eur J Immunol 6:882

Biron CA, Hutt-Fletcher LM, Wertz GT, Pagano JS (1981) Interferon induction and activation of non-specific effector cells by stimulation with lymphoblastoid cell lines in vitro. Int J Cancer 27:185–190

Blalock JE, Georgiades J, Johnson HM (1979) Immune-type interferon-induced transfer of viral resistance. J Immunol 122:1018–1021

Blanden RV, Gardner J (1976) The cell-mediated immune response to ectromelia virus infection. I. Kinetics and characteristics of the primary effector T cell response in vivo. Cell Immunol 22:271–282

Blazar B, Patarroyo M, Klein E, Klein G (1980) Increased sensitivity of human lymphoid lines to natural killer cells after induction of the Epstein-Barr viral cycle by superinfection or sodium butyrate. J Exp Med 151:614–627

Bro-Jorgensen K (1978) The interplay between lymphocytic choriomeningitis virus immune function and hemopoiesis in mice. Adv Virus Res 22:327–369

Ching C, Lopez C (1979) Natural killing of Herpes Simplex virus type-1 infected target cells: normal human responses and influence of antiviral antibody. Infect Immun 26:48–56

Cole GA, Nathanson N, Prendergast RA (1972) Requirement for Θ-bearing cells in lymphocytic choriomeningitis virus-induced central nervous system disease. Nature 238:335–337

Cole GA, Prendergast RA, Henney CS (1973) In vitro correlates of LCM virus-induced immune response. In: Lehmann-Grube F (ed) Lymphocytic choriomeningitis virus and other arenaviruses. Springer, Berlin Heidelberg New York, p 61

Cudkowicz G, Bennett M (1971) Peculiar immunobiology of bone marrow allografts. II. Rejection of parental grafts by resistant F1 hybrid mice. J Exp Med 134:1513–1528

Cudkowicz G, Lotzova E (1973) Hemopoietic cell-defined components of the major histocompatibility complex of mice: identification of responsive and unresponsive recipients for bone marrow transplants. Transplant Proc 54:1399–1405

Diamond RD, Keller R, Lee G, Finkel D (1977) Lysis of cytomegalovirus-infected human fibroblasts and transformed human cells by peripheral blood lymphoid cells from normal human donors. Proc Soc Exp Biol Med 154:259–263

Einhorn S, Blomgren H, Strander H (1978) Interferon and spontaneous cytotoxicity in man. II. Studies in patients receiving exogenous leukocyte interferon. Acta Med Scand 20:477–483

Gee SR, Clark DA, Rawls WE (1979) Differences between Syrian hamster strains in natural killer cell activity induced by infection with Pichinde virus. J Immunol 123:2618–2626

Gidlund M, Orn A, Wigzell H, Senik A, Gresser I (1978) Enhanced NK activity in mice injected with interferon and interferon inducers. Nature 273:759–761
Gilden DH, Cole GA, Nathanson N (1972) Immunopathogenesis of acute central nervous system disease produced by lymphocytic choriomeningitis virus. II. Adoptive immunization
of virus carriers. J Exp Med 135:874–889
Glimcher L, Shen FW, Cantor H (1977) Identification of a cell-surface antigen selectively expressed on the natural killer cell. J Exp Med 145:1–9
Greenberg SB, Six HR, Drake S, Couch RB (1979) Cell cytotoxicity due to specific influenza
antigen stimulation. Proc Natl Acad Sci USA 76:4622–4626
Greenberg SB, Criswell BS, Six HR, Couch RB (1980) Lymphocyte cytotoxicity to influenza virus-infected cells. II. Requirement for antibody and non-T lymphocytes. J Immunol 119:
2100–2106
Gresser I, Maury C, Brouty-Boye D (1972) Mechanism of the antitumor effect of interferon in
mice. Nature 239:167–168
Gresser I, Bandu MT, Brouty-Boyé D (1974) Interferon and cell division. IX. Interferon-resistant
L1210 cells: characteristics and origin. J Natl Cancer Inst 52:553–559
Grewal AS, Rouse BT, Babiuk LA (1977) Mechanisms of resistance to Herpes viruses: comparison of the effectiveness of different cell types in mediating antibody-dependent cell-mediated cytotoxicity. Infect Immun 15:698–703
Haller O, Wigzell H (1977) Suppression of natural killer cell activity with radioactive strontium:
effector cells are marrow dependent. J Immunol 118:1503–1506
Haller O, Kiessling R, Orn A, Wigzell H (1977) Generation of natural killer cells: an autonomous function of the bone marrow. J Exp Med 145:1411–1416
Hansson M, Kiessling R, Andersson B, Welsh RM (1980) Effect of interferon and interferon in-
ducers on the NK sensitivity of normal mouse thymocytes. J Immunol 125:2225–2531
Harfast B, Andersson T, Perlmann P (1975) Human lymphocyte cytotoxicity against mumps virus-infected target cells. J Immunol 114:1820–1823
Harfast B, Andersson T, Perlmann P (1978) Immunoglobulin-independent natural cytotoxicity
of Fc receptor – bearing human blood lymphocytes to mumps virus-infected target cells. J
Immunol 121:755–761
Harfast B, Andersson T, Alsheikly A, Perlmann P (1980a) Effect of Fc-receptor modulation on
mumps-virus dependent lymphocyte-mediated cytotoxicity in vitro. Scand J Immunol 11:
357–362
Harfast B, Orvell C, Alsheikly A, Andersson T (1980b) The role of viral glycoproteins in
mumps virus-dependent lymphocyte mediated cytotoxicity in vitro. Scand J Immunol 11:
391–400
Herberman RB, Nunn ME, Lavrin DH, Asofsky R (1973) Effect of antibody to theta antigen on
cell mediated immunity induced in syngeneic mice by murine sarcoma virus. J Natl Cancer
Inst 51:1509–1512
Herberman RB, Nunn ME, Lavrin DH (1975) Natural cytotoxic reactivity of mouse lymphoid
cells against syngeneic and allogeneic tumors. I. Distribution of reactivity and specificity.
Int J Cancer 16:216–229
Herberman RB, Nunn ME, Holden HT, Staal S, Djeu JY (1977) Augmentation of natural cyto-
toxic reactivity of mouse lymphoid cells against syngeneic and allogeneic target cells. Int J
Cancer 19:555–564
Herberman RB, Nunn ME, Holden HT (1978) Low density of Thy 1 antigen on mouse effector
cells mediating natural cytotoxicity against tumor cells. J Immunol 121:304–309
Herberman RB, Djeu JY, Kay HD, Ortaldo JR, Riccardi C, Bonnard GD, Holden HT, Fagnani
R, Santoni A, Puccetti P (1979) Natural killer cells: characteristics and regulation of activity.
Immunol Rev 44:43–70
Huddlestone J. Merigan TC, Oldstone MBA (1979) Induction and kinetics of natural killer cells
in humans following interferon therapy. Nature 282:417–419
Hutt-Fletcher LM, Gilbert CJ (to be published) Cytotoxic cells induced in vitro by Epstein-Barr
virus antigens.
Hutt LM, Huang YT, Dascomb HE, Pagano JS (1975) Enhanced destruction of lymphoid cell
lines by peripheral blood leukocytes taken from patients with acute infectious mononucleosis. J Immunol 115:243–248

Isaacs A, Lindenmann J (1957) Virus interference. I. The interferon. Proc R Soc Lond [Biol] 147:258–267

Ito M, Ralph P, Moore MAS (1980) Suppression of spleen natural killing activity induced by BCG. Clin Immunol Immunopathol 16:30–38

Jondal M, Targan S (1978) In vitro induction of cytotoxic effector cells with spontaneous killer cell specificity. J Exp Med 147:1621–1636

Jondal M, Spina C, Targan S (1978) Human spontaneous killer cells selective for tumor-derived target cells. Nature 272:62–64

Jones CL, Spindler KS, Holland JJ (1980) Studies on the tumorigenicity of cells persistently infected with vesicular stomatitis virus in nude mice. Virology 103:158–166

Karre K, Seeley JK (1979) Cytotoxic Thy 1.2 positive blasts with NK-like target selectivity in murine mixed lymphocyte cultures. J Immunol 123:1511–1518

Kasai M, LeClerc JC, McVay-Boudreau L, Shen FW, Cantor H (1979) Direct evidence that natural killer cells in nonimmune spleen cell populations prevent tumor growth in vivo. J Exp Med 149:1260–1264

Kiessling R, Welsh RM (1980) Killing of normal cells by activated mouse natural killer cells: evidence for two patterns of genetic regulation of lysis. Int J Cancer 25:611–615

Kiessling R, Wigzell H (1979) An analysis of the murine NK cell as to structure, function and biological relevance. Immunol Rev 44:165–208

Kiessling R, Klein E, Pross H, Wigzell H (1975a) "Natural" killer cells in the mouse. II. Cytotoxic cells with specificity for mouse Moloney leukemia cells characteristic of the killer cell. Eur J Immunol 5:117–121

Kiessling R, Klein E, Wigzell H (1975b) "Natural" killer cells in the mouse. I. Cytotoxic cells with specificity for mouse Moloney leukemia cells. Specificity and distribution according to genotype. Eur J Immunol 5:112–117

Kiessling R, Hochman PS, Haller O, Shearer GM, Wigzell H, Cudkowicz G (1977) Evidence for a similar or common mechanism for natural killer cell activity and resistance to hemopoietic grafts. Eur J Immunol 7:655–663

Kiessling R, Haller O, Fenyo EM, Steinitz M, Klein G (1978) Mouse natural killer (NK) cell activity against human cell lines is not influenced by superinfection of the target cell with xenotropic murine C-type virus. Int J Cancer 21:460–465

Kiessling R, Eriksson E, Hallenbeck LA, Welsh RM (1980) A comparative analysis of the cell surface properties of activated versus endogenous mouse natural killer cells. J Immunol 125:1551–1557

Kumar V, Bennett M (1976) Mechanisms of genetic resistance to Friend virus leukemia in mice. II. Resistance of mitogen-responsive lymphocytes mediated by marrow-dependent cells. J Exp Med 143:713–727

Kumar V, Bennett M, Eckner RJ (1974) Mechanisms of genetic resistance to Friend virus leukemia in mice. I. Role of [89]Sr-sensitive effector cells responsible for rejection of bone marrow allografts. J Exp Med 139:1093–1109

Kumar V, Caruso T, Bennett M (1976) Mechanism of genetic resistance to Friend virus leukemia. III. Susceptibility of mitogen responsive lymphocytes mediated by T cells. J Exp Med 143:728–740

Kumar V, Goldschmidt L, Eastcott JW, Bennett M (1978) Mechanisms of genetic resistance to Friend virus leukemia in mice. IV. Identification of a gene (FV-3) regulating immunosuppression in vitro, and its distinction from FV-2 and genes regulating marrow allograph reactivity. J Exp Med 147:422–433

Kumar V, Ben-Ezra J, Bennett M, Sonnenfield G (1979) Natural killer cells in mice treated with [89]Strontium: normal target-binding cell numbers but inability to kill even after interferon administration. J Immunol 123:1832–1838

Kuzumaki N, Koboyashi H (1976) Reduced transplantability of syngeneic mouse tumors superinfected with membrane viruses in Nu/Nu mice. Transplantation 22:545–550

Lam KM, Linna TJ (1979) Transfer of natural resistance to Marek's disease (JMV) with nonimmune spleen cells. I. Studies of cell population transferring resistance. Int J Cancer 24:662–667

Levy-Leblond E, Dupuy JM (1978) Neonatal susceptibility to MHV infection in mice. I. Transfer of resistance. J Immunol 118:1219–1222

Lopez C (1975) Genetics of natural resistance to Herpes virus infections in mice. Nature 258: 152–153

Lopez C (1978) Immunological nature of genetic resistance of mice to Herpes Simplex Type 1 infection. IARC 24:755–781

Lopez C, Bennett M (1978) Genetic resistance to HSV-1 in the mouse is mediated by a marrow (M)-dependent cell. Fourth International Congress for Virology, Center for Agricultural Publishing and Documentation, Wagenington, p 82

Lundstedt C (1969) Interaction between antigenically different cells. Virus-induced cytotoxicity by immune lymphoid cells in vitro. Acta Pathol Microbiol Scand 77:518–526

MacFarlan RI, Burns WH, White DO (1977) Two cytotoxic cells in peritoneal cavity of virus-infected mice: antibody-dependent macrophages and nonspecific killer cells. J Immunol 119: 1569–1574

MacFarlan RI, Ceredig R, White DO (1979) Comparison of natural killer cells induced by Kunjin virus and *Corynebacterium parvum* with those occurring in nude mice. Infect Immun 26: 832–836

Meguro H, Kervina M, Wright PF (1979) Antibody-dependent cell-mediated cytotoxicity against cells infected with respiratory syncitial virus: characterization of in vitro and in vivo properties. J Immunol 122:2521–2526

Merigan TC, Oldstone MBA, Welsh RM (1977) Interferon production during lymphocytic choriomeningitis virus infection of nude and normal mice. Nature 268:67–68

Minato N, Bloom BR, Jones C, Holland J, Reid LM (1979) Mechanism of rejection of virus persistently infected tumor cells by athymic nude mice. J Exp Med 149:1117–1133

Molomut N, Padnos M (1965) Inhibition of transplantable and spontaneous murine tumors by the M-P virus. Nature 208:948–950

Moore M, White WJ, Potter MR (1980) Modulation of target cell susceptibility to human natural killer cells by interferon. Int J Cancer 25:565–572

Nunn ME, Herberman RB, Holden HT (1977) Natural cell-mediated cytotoxicity in mice against non-lymphoid tumor cells and some normal cells. Int J Cancer 20:381–387

Odaka T, Matsukura M (1969) Inheritance of susceptibility to Friend mouse leukemia virus. VI. Reciprocal alteration of innate resistance or susceptibility by bone marrow transplantation between congenic strains. J Virol 4:837–843

Ojo E, Wigzell H (1978) Natural killer cells may be the only cells in normal mouse lymphoid populations endowed with cytolytic ability for antibody-coated tumor target cells. Scand J Immunol 7:297–306

Pape GR, Troye M, Axelsson B, Perlmann P (1979) Simultaneous occurrence of immunoglobulin dependent and independent mechanisms in natural cytotoxicity of human lymphocytes. J Immunol 122:2251–2260

Perrin LH, Zinkernagel RM, Oldstone MBA (1977) Immune response in humans after vaccination with vaccinia virus: generation of a virus specific cytotoxic activity by human peripheral lymphocytes. J Exp Med 146:949–969

Petranyi G, Kiessling R, Klein G (1975) Genetic control of "natural" killer lymphocytes in the mouse. Immuno Genet 2:53–61

Pfizenmaier K, Trostmann H, Rollinghoff M, Wagner H (1975) Temporary presence of self-reactive cytotoxic T lymphocytes during murine lymphocytic choriomeningitis. Nature 258: 238:240

Purtillo DT, DeFlorio D, Hutt LM, Bhawan J, Yang JPS, Otto R, Edwards W (1977) Variable phenotypic expression of an X-linked recessive lymphoproliferative syndrome. N Engl J Med 297:1077–1081

Quinnan GV, Manischewitz JE (1979) The role of natural killer cells and antibody-dependent cell-mediated cytotoxicity during murine cytomegalovirus infection. J Exp Med 150:1549–1554

Reid LM, Jones C, Holland J (1979) Virus carrier state suppresses tumorigenicity of tumor cells in athymic (nude) mice. J Gen Virol 42:609–614

Reid LM, Minato N, Bloom B, Holland J (to be published) Protection of virus persistently infected tumor cells and its implications for regulation of tumor growth and metastasis in athymic nude mice. Third International Symposium on Nude Mice

Riviere Y, Gresser I, Guillon JC, Tovey MG (1977) Inhibition by anti-interferon serum of lymphocytic choriomeningitis virus disease in suckling mice. Proc Nat Acad Sci USA 74:2135–2139

Rodda SJ, White DO (1976) Cytotoxic macrophages: a rapid nonspecific response to viral infection. J Immunol 117:2067–2072

Roder J, Duwe A (1979) The beige mutation in the mouse selectively impairs natural killer cell function. Nature 278:451–453

Santoli D, Trinchieri G, Lief FS (1978a) Cell-mediated cytotoxicity against virus-infected target cells in humans. I. Characterization of the effector lymphocyte. J Immunol 121:526–531

Santoli D, Trinchieri G, Koprowski H (1978b) Cell mediated cytotoxicity against virus-infected target cells in humans. II. Interferon induction and activation of natural killer cells. J Immunol 121(2):532–538

Savary CA, Lotzova E (1978) Suppression of natural killer cell cytotoxicity by splenocytes from *Corynebacterium parvum*-injected bone marrow – tolerant and infant mice. J Immunol 120:239–243

Schlager SI, Boyle MDP, Ohanian SH, Borsos T (1977) Effect of inhibiting DNA, RNA, and protein synthesis of tumor cells on their susceptibility to killing by antibody and complement. Cancer Res 37:1432–1437

Schlager SI, Ohanian SO, Borsos T (1978) Identification of lipids associated with the ability of tumor cells to resist humoral immune attack. J Immunol 120:472–480

Schreiber RD, Pangburn MK, Medicus RG, Muller-Eberhard HJ (1980) Raji cell injury and subsequent lysis by the purified cytolytic alternative pathway of human complement. Clin Immunol Immunopathol 15:384–396

Schroder EW, Merrick JM (1979) Alterations in glycosphingolipid patterns in a line of African Green monkey kidney cells infected with Herpesvirus. J Virol 32:734–740

Seeley JK, Golub SH (1978) Studies on cytotoxicity generated in human mixed lymphocyte cultures. I. Time course and target spectrum of several distinct concomitant cytotoxic activities. J Immunol 120:1415–1422

Seeley JK, Masucci G, Poros A, Klein E, Golub S (1979) Studies on cytotoxicity generated in human mixed lymphocyte cultures. II. Anti-K562 effectors are distinct from allospecific CTL and can be generated from NK-depleted T cells. J Immunol 123:1303–1311

Shope TC, Kaplan JPH (1979) Inhibition of the in vitro outgrowth of Epstein-Barr virus-infected lymphocytes by $T_G$ lymphocytes. J Immunol 123:2150–2155

Sissons JGP, Oldstone MBA (to be published) Antibody mediated destruction of virus infected cells. Adv Immunol 29:

Sullivan JL, Byron KS, Brewster FE, Purtillo DT (1980) Deficient natural killer cell activity in the X-linked lymphoproliferative syndrome. Science 210:543–544

Svedmyr EA, Jondal M (1975) Cytotoxic effector cells specific for B cell lines transferred by Epstein-Barr virus are present in patients with infectious mononucleosis. Proc Natl Acad Sci USA 72:1622–1626

Svedmyr EA, Deinhardt F, Klein G (1974) Sensitivity of different target cells to the killing action of peripheral lymphocytes stimulated by autologous lymphoblastical cell lines. Int J Cancer 13:891–903

Tai A, Burton RC, Warner NL (1980) Differential natural killer cell reactivity against T cell lymphomas by cells from normal or stimulated mice. J Immunol 124:1705–1711

Talmadge JE, Meyers KM, Prieur DJ, Starkey JR (1980a) Role of NK cells in tumor growth and metastasis in beige mice. Nature 284:622–624

Talmadge JE, Meyers KM, Prieur DJ, Starkey JR (1980b) Role of natural killer cells in tumor growth and metastasis: normal and beige mice. J Natl Cancer Inst 65:929–935

Tardieu M, Hery C, Dupuy JM (1980) Neonatal susceptibility to $MHV_3$ infection in mice. II. Role of natural effector marrow cells in transfer of resistance. J Immunol 124:418–423

Thorley-Lawson DA, Chess L, Strominger JL (1977) Suppression of in vitro Epstein-Barr virus infection – a new role for adult human T lymphocytes. J Exp Med 146:495–508

Timonen T (1979) Human natural cell-mediated cytotoxicity against fetal fibroblasts. IV. Comparison of cytotoxic activity with antibody-dependent cell-mediated cytotoxicity. Scand J Immunol 9:239–245

Traub E (1936) Persistence of lymphocytic choriomeningitis virus in immune animals and its relation to immunity. J Exp Med 63:847–861

Trinchieri G, Santoli D (1978) Anti-viral activity induced by culturing lymphocytes with tumor-derived or virus-transformed cells. Enhancement of natural killer cell activity by interferon and antagonistic inhibition of susceptibility of target cells to lysis. J Exp Med 147:1314–1333

Trinchieri G, Santoli D, Dee RR, Knowles BB (1978) Anti-viral activity induced by culturing lymphocytes with tumor-derived or virus-transformed cells. Identification of the anti-viral activity as interferon and characterization of the human effector lymphocyte subpopulation. J Exp Med 124:1299–1313

Volkert M, Larsen JH, Pfau CJ (1964) Studies on immunological tolerance to LCM virus. 4. The question of immunity in adoptively immunized virus carriers. Acta Pathol Microbiol Scand 61:268–282

Welsh RM (1978a) Mouse natural killer cells: induction, specificity, and function. J Immunol 121:1631–1635

Welsh RM (1978b) Cytotoxic cells induced during lymphocytic choriomeningitis virus infection of mice. I. Characterization of natural killer cell induction. J Exp Med 148:163–181

Welsh RM, Doe WF (1980) Cytotoxic cells induced during lymphocytic choriomeningitis virus infection of mice. III. Natural killer cell activity in cultured spleen leukocytes concomitant with T cell dependent immune interferon production. Infect Immun 30:473–483

Welsh RM, Hallenbeck LA (1980) Effect of virus infections on target cell susceptibility to natural killer cell mediated lysis. J Immunol 124:2491–2497

Welsh RM, Kiessling RW (1980) Natural killer cell response to lymphocytic choriomeningitis virus in beige mice. Scand J Immunol 11:363–367

Welsh RM, Pfau CJ (1972) Determinants of lymphocytic choriomeningitis interference. J Gen Virol 14:177–187

Welsh RM, Zinkernagel RM (1977) Hetero-specific cytotoxic cell activity induced during the first three days of acute lymphocytic choriomeningitis virus infection in mice. Nature 268: 646–648

Welsh RM, Zinkernagel RM, Hallenbeck LA (1979) Cytotoxic cells induced during lymphocytic choriomeningitis virus infection of mice. II. Specificities of the natural killer cells. J Immunol 122:475–481

Welsh RM, Karre K, Hansson M, Kunkel LA, Kiessling R (1981) Interferon-mediated protection of normal and tumor target cells against lysis by mouse natural killer cells. J Immunol 126:219–225

Wheelock EF, Sibley WA (1964) Interferon in human serum during clinical virus infections. Lancet 2:382–385

Wong CY, Woodruff JJ, Woodruff JF (1977) Generation of cytotoxic T lymphocytes during Coxsackie virus B-3 infection. III. Role of sex. J Immunol 119:591–597

Yamada T, Hatano M (1972) Lowered transplantability of cultured tumor cells by persistent infection with paramyxovirus. Jpn J Cancer Res 63:647–655

Young WW, Hakamori S, Durdik JM, Henney CS (1980) Identification of ganglio-N-tetraosyl-ceramide as a new cell surface marker for murine natural killer (NK) cells. J Immunol 124: 199–201

Zarling JM, Bach FH (1978) Sensitization of lymphocytes against pooled allogeneic cells. I. Generation of cytotoxicity against autologous human lymphoblastoid cell lines. J Exp Med 147:1334–1340

Zarling JM, Nowinski RC, Bach FH (1975) Lysis of leukemia cells by spleen cells of normal mice. Proc Nat Acad Sci USA 72:2780–2784

Zinkernagel RM, Doherty PC (1974) Restriction of in vitro T cell mediated cytotoxicity in lymphocytic choriomeningitis within a syngeneic or semiallogeneic system. Nature 248:701–702

Zinkernagel RM, Welsh RM (1976) H-2 compatibility requirement for virus-specific T cell mediated effector functions in vivo. I. Specificity of T cells confering antiviral protection against lymphocytic choriomeningitis virus is associated with H-2K and H-2D. J Immunol 117:1495–1502

# Surveillance of Primitive Cells by Natural Killer Cells

ROLF KIESSLING* AND HANS WIGZELL**

## 1 Introduction

Natural killer cells (NK cells) were originally described and defined as a distinct group of cells using in vitro cytolytic assays against malignant cells (*Kiessling* et al. 1975a; *Herberman* et al. 1975b). The fact that the NK cells constitute such a recent discovery may in part be due to the previous prevailing focus in tumor immunology requiring strict specificity of an immune reaction to allow a proper interest. It is now clear that NK cells are cells able to endow the individual with immune capacity, that is, to exclude the occurrence of certain diseases. However, it is equally clear that the specificity patterns expressed by NK cells are of a "broader" type than is displayed by T or B lymphocytes against conventional antigens. Still, little doubt exists that NK cells do indeed express a distinct selectivity in their lytic and binding patterns (*Kiessling* et al. 1975). The specific profile as to lysis is in fact one of the best accepted markers for NK cells, since natural killer cells have very few markers on their surface which define the lytic cell being studied as an NK cell (*Kiessling* and *Wigzell* 1979).

   Natural killer cells constitute a cell type on their own on the basis of several parameters. They can be shown to be different from classical B and T lymphocytes as well as monocytes and macrophages (*Kiessling* et al. 1975). Yet, enriched populations of NK cells display morphologic features that have allowed most workers to consider them to be lymphocytes (*Roder* et al. 1978; *Saksela* et al. 1979). Whether the natural killer cells can be considered to be a kind of pre-B or -T lymphocyte has attracted intense interest and studies over the last few years. It is clear, however, that individuals lacking conventional T and B lymphocytes can be shown to display normal NK levels (*Pross* et al. 1979; *Kiessling* et al. 1975b), whereas bone marrow diseases or destruction will lead to a rapid decay in NK activity (*Haller* and *Wigzell* 1977; *Seaman* et al. 1979). Certain surface markers normally associated with T lymphocytes have also been found on NK cells (*Herberman* et al. 1978; *Herberman* et al. 1979), but this does not, according to our view, justify any claims at pres-

*Dept. of Tumor Biology, Karolinska Institute, S-104 01 Stockholm, Sweden
**Dept. of Immunology, Uppsala University Biomedical Center, Box 582, S-571 23 Uppsala, Sweden

ent that NK cells indeed are pre-T cells. Actual demonstration of differentiation from NK to T cell functions would be required, in this case requiring clones of cells in the assay.

In the present review we have taken a personal view on natural killer cells as to in vivo relevance and specificity, both with regard to malignant cells and with regard to possible regulation of normal functions or resistance towards infections. This review is by no means complete and does merely represent our considerations of some select questions in relation to the biologic relevance of the NK cells. Readers interested in more diversified reviews on NK cells should study in particular a recent collection of such articles (*Möller* 1979).

## 2 In Vivo Relevance of NK Cells in Relation to Tumors

It is notable that the reason why NK cells originally created so much interest is due to their possible involvement as a T-cell-independent immune surveillance mechanism against tumor growth (*Chernyakhovskaya* et al. 1970). Subsequently, however, they have also been implied as possible effector cells in rejection of virus-infected cells and in regulation of normal cell stem cell differentiation (*Welsh* and *Zinkernagel* 1977; *Kiessling* et al. 1977; *Reid* et al. 1979).

Several lines of evidence of a more indirect nature argue for the involvement of NK

Table 1. Evidence for in vivo relevance of mouse NK cells in rejection of tumor cells

---

1. Strong positive correlation between in vitro NK activity and in vivo tumor resistance in rejection studies of tumor transplants in various genotypes (*Kiessling* et al. 1975c; *Sendo* et al. 1975).
2. T-cell deficient $F_1$ hybrid mice have an increased resistance to the growth of an NK-sensitive semisyngeneic lymphoma (*Kiessling* et al. 1976).
3. NK-sensitive tumors grow less well in nude mice than normal littermates (*Kiessling* et al. 1976; *Warner* et al. 1977).
4. B-cell deprived mice have elevated NK activity and are better able to resist NK-sensitive, syngeneic tumors (*Brodt* and *Gordon*, to be published).
5. Lymphocytes enriched for NK cells efficiently delay tumor growth upon transfer into irradiated syngeneic recipients (*Kasai* et al. 1979; *Kiessling* et al. 1976).
6. Bone marrow chimeras between NK high- or low-reactive $F_1$ genotypes show the same in vivo resistance to semisyngeneic tumor transplant as the bone marrow donor strain (*Haller* et al. 1977).
7. Newly hatched chickens can be passively protected against Marek's disease and leukemia induction by transfer of an "NK-like" cell type from adult animal (*Lam* and *Juhani* 1979).
8. Good correlation between in vitro NK activity and the ability to reject prelabeled tumor cells in a 4-h in vivo assay (*Rickard* et al. 1980).
9. Aging mice (> 6 months) exhibit a marked decline in NK-mediated tumor rejection in vivo or in vitro (*Haller* et al. 1977) and an increasing incidence of spontaneous tumors.
10. The mouse mutant beige, selectively impaired in NK function (*Roder* and *Duwe* 1979), rejects tumor transplants and metastasis less efficient (*Kärre* et al. 1980; *Talmadge* et al. 1980).
11. Humans, carrying the analogous beige gene (Chediak-Higashi gene) are selectively impaired in NK function and exhibit a profound (85%) incidence of a spontaneous, "lymphoma-like" lymphoproliferative disorder (*Roder* et al. 1980).

---

cells in rejection of transplantable tumors. These are listed in Table 1 and will therefore not be discussed here in detail. They include a number of correlations between in vitro NK activity and in vivo rejection potential against a small tumor inocula of the same tumor as used in the NK assay. The correlation was originally noted in the genetic regulation of in vitro activity and in vivo tumor resistance studying a variety of different semi-syngeneic $F_1$ hybrids (*Petranyi* et al. 1975). A similar age dependency between in vitro NK activity and in vivo tumor resistance has also been observet with a NK-sensitive tumor line (*Haller* et al. 1977). The correlation studies between NK activity and in vivo resistance have all been carried out using long-term transplantation assays. Although the transplantation resistance in some of these systems clearly was T-cell independent (*Kiessling* et al. 1976; *Warner* et al. 1977), one cannot critically exclude the participation of several other types of T-dependent and -independent host resistance factors. As an example, it could be mentioned that *Chow* et al. (1979) characterized the "natural" T-independent rejection of some syngeneic tumors as not being due to NK cells, but probably macrophages or natural antibodies. It is therefore of importance to analyze the relative importance of NK cells versus other host resistance factors in each tumor-host system studied. One way of doing this has been to use alternatives to the conventional transplantation rejection assays. Two such experimental systems in which one can more precisely analyze the cell population active in growth retardation of tumors deserves mentioning. First, successful attempts to analyze NK activity in a "semi-in vivo" system using the so-called Winn assay has now been described by several groups. Originally the importance of NK cells in conferring resistance to the outgrowth of a tumor inoculum by passive admixture with spleen cells depleted of T-cells, B-cells, or monocytes and enriched for NK cells was observed with the MuLV-induced lymphoma YAC (*Kiessling* et al. 1976). The same method was recently also employed by another group, who by positive selection of NK cells using alloantisera, such as Ly-5 (*Kasai* et al. 1979), could show more conclusively that NK cells are active in conferring resistance to tumor growth in Winn assays. The advantage with the Winn assay method is that it allows a direct comparison of a particular cell fraction, both with regard to in vitro cytotoxicity and in vivo tumor growth retardation. On the other hand, it is clearly a very "artificial" in vivo model, since it involves premixing of effector cells and tumor cells prior to local inoculation.

The systemic administration of cell populations varying in their NK potential injected into NK-depleted hosts appears as a somewhat more valid in vivo model. Thus *Lam* and *Linna* demonstrated that resistance to the avian malignancy Marek's disease in chickens could be transferred with spleen cells from nonimmunized, adult, resistant chickens to newly hatched susceptible ones. The cells transferring resistance did not belong to the major T-cell, B-cell, or macrophage populations and therefore bore some resemblance to the NK cell as described in murine and human systems (*Lam* and *Linna* 1979). This adoptive transfer system may well be the very first one to demonstrate the in vivo relevance of NK cells in primary oncogenesis. Recently, *Riccardi* and co-workers (1981) used and adoptive transfer system to study murine NK cells. These authors demonstrated that treatment of mice with cyclophosphamide (Cy) caused a marked depression both of in vitro NK activity and in vivo natural reactivity against intravenous challenge with [125]IUdR-labeled tumor cells. The ability of passively transferred normal spleen cells to reconstitute such mice correlated well with levels of NK activity of donor cells with regard to several different parameters such as organ and strain distribution, age regulation, and cell surface characteristics of the active cell type. This model would thus seem close to ideal for analyzing factors relating to the regulation and differentiation of NK cells.

It remains to be demonstrated, however, to what extent this assay could be valid also for analyzing the role of NK cells in long-term transplantation assays, since the NK depressive effect of cyclophosphamide on the host will wane after 6–8 days. This "early" period after tumor inoculation, however, may well be very critical for NK "surveillance". In fact, *Hanna* and *Fiddler* recently have shown that a single injection of Cy 4 days before tumor cell inoculation significantly enhanced the formation of pulmonary and extrapulmonary metastasis (*Hanna* and *Fiddler* 1980). Reconstitution of Cy-treated recipients with syngeneic lymphoid cells from normal mice reversed the effects of Cy. Again, the active cell bore many of the characteristics of an NK cell, since it was nonadherent, resistant to treatment with anti-theta serum, and Cy sensitive.

These studies altogether would then suggest that NK cells might be of importance in host defense against metastatic spread of tumor cells. Further support for this concept of NK cells as active against metastatic spread of tumor cells comes from *Gorelik* et al. (1979), who observed that cell lines established from metastatic foci have a decreased sensitivity for NK cells compared to cells from the primary tumor, as would be predicted if NK cells exert negative selection on the tumor population in vivo. Finally, as will be discussed, the beige model has also supported the role of NK cells in acting against metastatic spread.

Another approach of transferring high NK reactivity to low reactive recipients was accomplished in a system studying long-term transplantation assays by *Haller* et al. (1977). Here, we produced radiation chimeras by inoculation of fetal liver or bone marrow into lethally irradiated recipients, and found that the degree of in vitro NK activity as well as resistance to challenge with an NK-sensitive lymphoma in vivo was dependent on the NK reactivity of the bone marrow donor mice. From these experiments we concluded that the degree of NK reactivity seems to be dictated by bone marrow stem cells and also that the growth of a transplantable lymphoma was influenced by the in vitro NK activity of the bone marrow donors. This data thus strongly argued for the role of NK cells in rejection of transplantable lymphomas, particularly since the experiments were performed in T-cell-deficient animals. One cannot entirely exclude from these experiments, however, that other T-cell-independent host resistance factors with a similar genetic control as the NK system may be involved as well.

A totally different approach in looking at the in vivo involvement of NK cells in tumor rejection is to ask whether tumors displaying high sensitivity to NK lysis in vitro would be more easily rejected than the resistant ones when injected in vivo into syngeneic animals. Evidence that this may indeed be true has been obtained in several independent studies. Two examples could be mentioned. *Warner* et al., working with lymphoid tumors of Balb/c origin, found that only those tumor cell lines lysed in vitro by NK cells showed a reduced growth rate in syngeneic nude mice known to be highly NK reactive compared to their heterozygous litter mates. It could also be shown that tumor cell lines which were resistant to in vitro lysis did not show this reduced in vivo growth rate in syngeneic nude mice (*Warner* et al. 1977). Also in a more recent report from our laboratory (*Riesenfeld* et al. 1980), a similar correlation between in vitro NK susceptibility and in vivo growth pattern was seen. This system was comprised of two AKR lymphomas with a similar growth pattern but with significant differences in vitro with regard to susceptibility to NK-mediated lysis. These tumor cells were grafted into AKRxCBA F1 hybrids which had been lethally irradiated and then protected with bone marrow of CBA (high NK) or AKR (low NK) origin and which displayed high or low NK levels if coming from CBA and AKR donors, respectively. We found the in vivo growth pattern of the two AKR lymphomas to be correlated in a strikingly positive manner with the NK activities of the recipients. Thus, high NK activity in the recipients resulted in a significant increase in resistance toward the outgrowth of the NK-sensitive AKR lymphoma but had only marginal impact on the relatively NK-resistant lymphoma. This was true irrespective of whether the recipients were thymectomized before marrow reconstitution. Again, this system would thus further suggest an important role for NK cells in mediating in vivo resistance toward NK-susceptible tumors.

One important question when trying to compare the in vivo growth of NK sensitive versus insensitive tumors is to decide what levels of sensitivity one should regard as significant in classifying a tumor as "NK insensitive". There are reasons to believe that low levels (less than 10% lysis) of sensitivity for NK lysis could also be of in vivo relevance. It can in fact be questioned whether any tumor target can be regarded as completely resistant to NK lysis, given the optimal conditions for the system. To cite an example, using highly activated NK cells obtained, for example, by virus activation, cell lines which are normally resistant to lysis by "endogenous" NK cells are also killed to a significant degree [as is the case with, e.g., the mouse L-cell line or the P 815 tumor target (*Welsh* and *Zinkernagel* 1977)].

There are some examples where NK cells seem also to be active in vivo against targets of low sensitivity. This has been indicated by the positive genetic correlation also noted between NK reactivity and in vivo tumor resistance when tumors of low NK sensitivity are used. Thus the H-2-linked resistance factor was noted both in vivo and in vitro when the relatively NK-insensitive tumor EL-4 was used (*Harmon* et al. 1977; *Klein* et al. 1978). Also, the YAC system could serve to illustrate this point. Here, the YAC ascites tumor shows relatively low sensitivity for NK lysis compared to the YAC-1 in vitro line (*Kiessling* et al. 1975a). In order to obtain the same tumor incidence, 100-fold more YAC-1 cells than YAC ascites cells were used, but even at this high cell dose the same genotype dependence was noted for the YAC-1 in vitro line as for low cell dose of the ascites cells (*Kiessling* et al. 1975c). This result would be in concert with the view that YAC-1 cells express more of the relevant target structure than do YAC ascites cells but that the amount expressed in the ascites cells would be enough to make these cells ultimately sensitive for NK-mediated in vivo rejection. A final point to be mentioned in this context is the in vivo relevance of the low levels of sensitivity for NK lysis that have also been noted for normal, nonmalignant cells of hematopoietic origin. Since there is now evidence that NK cells can be active also in rejection of bone marrow grafts in vivo, as will be discussed, this could serve as a last example of the possible in vivo relevance of even low levels of target cell susceptibility for NK lysis. In conclusion, since it seems that the classification of target cells in the NK system into sensitive or insensitive often is more relative than absolute, studies to correlate in vitro sensitivity for lysis and in vivo rejectability must be designed in such a way that they may detect such relative differences.

We have here reviewed some examples of how various experimental manipulations, such as genetic crosses in the parent to F1 model or depletion-passive reconstitution experiments have provided indirect evidence for NK cells being active in rejecting or retarding tumor growth. It would be of considerable advantage, however, if a less artificial experimental model could be used where the result of a syngeneic tumor challenge could be studied in a nonmanipulated host selectively devoid of NK activity. There is now much hope in that such a model has become available through recent studies of immune functions of the C57Black mutant beige[J] (bg). From the original studies of *Roder* and *Duwe* (1979) homozygosity for the bg allele leads to severe impairment of NK activity, whereas other types of cell-mediated immunity, such as tumor killing by activated macrophages, as well as B- and T-cell functions are intact (*Roder* et al. 1979a). Will the beige model provide us with the final answer to whether NK cells are active in immune surveillance against neoplasia? At this moment there are a number of laboratories working with the beige model in studies of tumor resistance as well as in studies involving some of the other proposed in vivo activities of NK cells, including their role in defense against virus infections and as a rejection mechanism against normal bone marrow grafts. Within a short time we will, therefore, have the answer to many important questions relating to the in vivo relevance of NK cells. How conclusive will the beige model be for our understanding of NK cells? There are some disadvantages with this model which should be mentioned.

First, the beige mutation has several other phenotypic manifestations apart from its effect on the NK system. It was originally described because of its affect on lysosomal membrane functions, including abnormal granulocyte morphology and functions, as well as melanosomal function, leading to the light "beige" coat color (*Gallin* et al. 1974; *Windhorst* and *Padgett* 1973). It could therefore be asked to what extent these manifestations will also affect the outcome of induced or spontaneous oncogenesis. Secondly, beige mice are not totally devoid of NK activity. This is most clearly apparent after a strong induction of NK activity, e.g., by an acute infection with lymphocytic choriomeningitis virus (LCMV), where considerable levels of NK activity can be seen (up to 25% lysis against the YAC-1 lymphoma), although they are still less reactive than the LCMV-boostered +/bg controls (*Welsh* and *Kiessling* 1980). Thus, the beige mutation leads to more of a relative than a total defect of the NK system, which would seem to make this animal model somewhat less ideal in studying NK functions than the nude mutation with its striking impairment of T-cell maturation has been for analyzing T-cell functions. Nevertheless, there are some clear advantages with this model as compared to some of the previously discussed experimental systems. First, it offers a possibility to study the effect of very low NK activity on an NK highly reactive background strain, why beige mice should therefore not merely be regarded as yet another NK low reactive strain. Secondly, the low reactivity of the beige mice is stable throughout their entire lifespan (*Roder* and *Duwe* 1979), which makes this model clearly superior to most of those involving the manipulative suppression of NK activity, e.g., by cyclophosphamide or [89]Sr which only temporarily decreases NK activity. In fact, this stability of low reactivity is an absolute prerequisite for studying the outcome of long-term transplantation assays or, even more important, for experiment with induced or spontaneous oncogenesis which may require at least several months of observation.

Having these limitations and advantages with the beige model in mind, we would like to briefly summarize the currently available information on tumor resistance in beige mice. First, results from our group (*Kärre* et al. 1980) as well as from that of *Talmadge* et al. (1980) have clearly demonstrated that this mouse mutant is less resistant to the growth of a small inoculum of transplantable tumors than are the bg/+ control mice. In our study this was demonstrated with two syngeneic C57Bl/lymphomas (EL-4 and P-52), where a clear difference in tumor take as well as latency period was apparent for both of these tumor lines when comparing the bg/bg mice with the +/bg littermates. One point which should be emphasized is the observation that this difference was most apparent in the early phases of tumor growth, while later it became less clear, although it still remained significant throughout the observation period. Again this would stress the importance of NK defense in the early phases of tumor surveillance, a fact further supported by applying a technique studying the rapid clearance (6–18 h) of $^{125}$IUdR-labeled tumor cells in beige mice. The application of this technique for measuring NK activity in vivo was originally developed by *Riccardi* et al. (1980), who demonstrated that the clearance of i.v.-injected IUdR-labeled tumor cells correlated well with the level of host NK activity. When this assay was applied to the beige model, we found that NK-sensitive lymphomas were cleared at a significantly lower rate, both when counting whole body clearance as well as spleen and lung clearance (*Kärre* et al. 1980).

We have already discussed some indications that NK cells may be of importance in conferring resistance to metastatic spread. The beige model further substantiated this idea. Thus *Talmadge* et al. (1980) demonstrated with the B16 melanoma cell not only an increased growth rate but also an increased metastatic potential in bg/bg mice compared to +/bg controls.

In conclusion, there is now definite evidence that beige mice are indeed less resistant to the growth and metastatic spread of some syngeneic transplantable tumors. Within the limitations of the beige model, this would strongly support the concept which has emerged from the previously discussed experimental models that NK cells can act as an early rejection mechanism against a small inoculum of tumor cells. Although the ability of mice to rapidly reject a small inoculum of transplantable tumors would appear as a reasonable model to study "immune surveillance" against a newly arisen neoplastic clone, the use of transplantable tumors can clearly not be taken as a final evidence for the involvement of NK cells in the prevention of primary or induced oncogenesis. Several laboratories are now involved in extensive studies of the incidence of induced and spontaneous lymphomas in beige mice, but at the moment of writing no definite answer has yet been provided. Much of this interest of the beige model has been stirred by the observation that humans homozygous for the Chediak-Higashi (CH) gene, as analogue to the mouse beige gene, have a profound increase in spontaneous lymphoproliferative malignancy (*Dent* et al. 1966). These patients also show a severely depressed NK lytic activity (*Roder* et al. 1980).

In a very preliminary note, *Loutit* et al. (1980) reported a high incidence (27%) of disseminating lymphoma in a relatively small group of mice carrying the beige gene. Although this study remains to be extended to a more definite report involving larger groups of mice, histology of the tumors, and appropriate heterozygous controls, it may well be the first indications that NK cells are one of the major factors involved in control of oncogenesis.

# 3 The Specificity of NK Cells

Whereas general agreement exists that natural killer cells can kill several different malignant cell lines with distinct histogenetic origins, controversy does still reside as to the fine specificity of NK cells. Likewise, the issue is still not settled whether NK cells in a given individual all express the same specificity or whether they may express individually specific, clonally distributed receptors of varying specificity. In our own studies in the murine system we have failed to find any evidence for such a clonal variability in specificity of NK cells (for discussion on this point see *Kiessling* and *Wigzell* 1979), but reports claiming such a heterogeneity pattern have been coming forth in studies of mouse as well as human natural killer cells (*Herberman* et al. 1975a; *Jensen* and *Koren* 1979). Likewise, it is not clear whether several different features at the target level such as hydrophobicity, charge, and varying glycolipid-glycoprotein patterns all add up to give "NK-specificity" or if there indeed exist unique NK-target structures that can be defined at the macromolecular level explaining this selectivity of binding and lysis by NK cells, as suggested by the finding of *Roder* et al. (1979b). In this review we will concentrate to a major degree on the specificity of natural killer cells in relation to the degree of differentiation of the target cell. We will do this since a series of independent observations have led us to the conclusion that NK cells very often would seem to be particularly prone to act in an aggressive manner against cells at an "embryonic" or early stage in their respective differentiation.

After having defined that many in vitro growing malignant cell lines were susceptible to NK lysis (*Kiessling* et al. 1975a), a first indication that normal primitive cell types may also be sensitive for NK cells was noted in relation to bone marrow stem cells. In a parallel analysis it was thus possible to show that resistance in an individual to bone marrow grafting in the s.c. hybrid resistance of the mouse (*Cudkowicz* 1968) was in many ways displaying identical features with NK activity (*Kiessling* et al. 1977).

These results have since been extended in the murine system in particular by *Cudkowicz* and co-workers (see parallel article in this volume), and good data do now exist strongly indicating the NK cells as participants in such a rejection system in vivo.

Recent data with human marrow cells as targets for NK lysis in vitro further support the concept of increased lytic susceptibility of "embryonic" versus "adult" cells of a similar type (*Hansson* et al. 1981). Using human peripheral blood NK cells with increased lytic activity after interferon activation it was thus found that human marrow cells to a significant degree can be lyzed by these NK cells (Table 2). This was particularly clear when the marrow was derived from human fetuses (16–19 weeks of gestation), with the fetal marrow cells being on the average twice as sensitive (expressed as percentage specific lysis) as their adult counterparts. It is not clear whether this represents an average increased sensitivity of the fetal marrow cells per se or, as would seem more likely, the fetal marrow contains a higher percentage of a particular NK-susceptible target type. Preli-

Table 2. Susceptibility of primary fetal or adult bone marrow cells and fetal thymocytes to normal and Interferon-activated NK cells (*Hansson* et al. 1981)

| Target cells | Number of experiments | Treatment of effector cells | % lysis + S.D.[a] at effector/target ratio of | | |
|---|---|---|---|---|---|
| | | | 50:1 | 25:1 | 12:1 |
| Adult bone marrow | 12 | – | $6.5 \pm 4.8$ | $5.0 \pm 3.7$ | $4.2 \pm 2.6$ |
| | 9 | IF | $13.7 \pm 8.4$ | $12.6 \pm 6.9$ | $9.1 \pm 6.3$ |
| Fetal bone marrow | 6 | – | $18.3 \pm 6.8$ | $16.3 \pm 4.5$ | $9.0 \pm 1.8$ |
| | 4 | IF | $31.3 \pm 6.7$ | $26.3 \pm 3.7$ | $19.9 \pm 2.1$ |
| Fetal thymocytes | 3 | – | $25.3 \pm 14.5$ | $25.1 \pm 8.7$ | $15.4 \pm 2.9$ |
| | 3 | IF | $39.3 \pm 13.4$ | $33.2 \pm 9.8$ | $27.5 \pm 6.1$ |

[a] Mean values $\pm$ S.D. from a pool of experiments

minary data (*Hansson* et al., to be published) indicating that the colony-forming cells of the marrow are included among such NK cells are in line with such reasonings.

In yet another system it has been demonstrated that a similar positive correlation between NK susceptibility and the less differentiated stage of the target cells may exist, namely within the thymocyte populations (*Nunn* et al. 1977; *Hansson* et al. 1979a). After the initial observation that the murine thymus contains some cells with NK susceptibility it was noted that there was a striking strain restriction in this display pattern, where high NK strains would display low susceptibility in the thymus for NK lysis and conversely for low NK strains (*Hansson* et al. 1979a). Age was furthermore shown to be highly important and only young mice contained thymocytes with a high percentage of NK-susceptible targets. A more detailed analysis of the thymocytes susceptible to NK attack yielded results suggesting that the target was a cortical, relatively large cell with additional features indicating the cell to be of quite immature type (*Hansson* et al. 1979b). Recently, data in the human have produced results in line with these conclusions, as fetal human thymocyte populations could be shown to be highly susceptible to NK lysis (*Hansson* et al. 1981, see also Table 2) in a manner significantly different from the relatively resistant behavior of adult human thymus cells as reported by others (*Ohno* et al. 1977).

Parallel studies using cloned, malignant cells have yielded independent confirmation for the concept that "embryonic" tumor targets are more susceptible to NK lysis than their more "differentiated" counterparts. This was initially suggested by studies which used murine embryonal carcinoma cells and compared them to differentiated endodermal teratocarcinoma lines (*Stern* et al. 1980). Here it could be shown that the embryonal carcinoma cells as a group constituted a highly NK susceptible population, whereas among the endodermal teratomas several were found to be highly NK resistant. Since embryonal carcinoma cells lacking major histocompatibility (MHC) antigens were found to be highly susceptible to NK cells while in parallel no lytic impact on these cells were demonstrable using cytolytic T cells (*Stern* et al. 1980), this would further add to the exclusion of MHC structures as participating as a target unit for NK lysis (*Becker* et al. 1976). The fact that the embryonal carcinoma cells lacking MHC were totally resistant, even when attempting T-killer cell lines in combination with glueing lectins, would on the other hand suggest that MHC-derived molecules may not only code for dominating target structures for the antigen-binding receptors for T lymphocytes but could also serve as a decisive lytic target unit for the actual lysis mediated by such cells.

In order to further refine the system, experiments were also performed using tumor cell lines of known NK susceptibility, which were then induced to differentiate in vitro under controlled conditions. We carried out experiments both in human (K562, U937 as target cells) or murine (Friend DBA/2 leukemia cells) systems yielding essentially identical results. In short, parallel with induced differentiation [showing itself in the various systems according to the lineage of the tumor target analyzed, e.g., glycophorin and hemoglobin production in K562 (*Andersson* et al. 1979)], induction of ADCC ability, and Fc receptors for IgG in the U937 line (*Koren* et al. 1979), there was a reduction of significant amplitude with regard to NK susceptibility. In some experiments advantage was also taken of the presence of naturally occurring cloned variants from the K562 line with a "spontaneous" higher stage of differentiation. Again, such variants displayed the increased resistance towards NK lysis. Table 3 summarizes the results of the various normal and tumor systems. It would seem clear that cells undergoing differentiation may frequently move from a NK-susceptible phase into one of resistance. Competition experiments in

Table 3. Evidence that cells within the same lineage are more susceptible to NK lysis in their early stages of differentiation

---

*Normal cells*
a) Thymocytes: Cortical thymocytes contain a fraction of cells susceptible to NK lysis. These cells have all hallmarks of being "immature" cells (*Hansson* et al. 1979[b]). Fetal mouse and human thymocytes are more susceptible to NK lysis than adult thymocytes (*Hansson* et al. 1981; *Hansson* et al. 1979).
b) Bone marrow cells: Human bone marrow contains a fraction of cells susceptible to NK lysis (*Hansson* et al. 1981). This fraction would seem to contain the stem cells forming colonies in vitro (*Hansson* et al., to be published). Fetal human marrow is approximately twice as susceptible to NK lysis than are adult bone marrow cells (*Hansson* et al. 1981).

*Malignant cells*
a) Teratomas: Embryonal murine carcinoma cells are NK susceptible, whereas endodermal teratocarcinomas stemming from such embryonal carcinoma cells are resistant (*Stern* et al. 1980). Controlled differentiation of an embryonal carcinoma line in vitro results in significant reduction in NK susceptibility (*Stern* et al., to be published).
b) Erythroid leukemia: The human K562 line is highly susceptible to NK lysis. In vitro induced or spontaneous differentiation is always accompanied with reduction in NK susceptibility (*Gidlund* et al., to be published). Likewise, Friend-virus-induced murine leukemia cells undergoing in vitro induced differentiation lose their NK susceptibility (*Gidlund* et al., unpublished work).
c) Histiocytoma: The human U937 line is highly NK susceptible and lacks Fc receptors and ADCC ability. In vitro induced differentiation will result in appearance of Fc receptors and development of ADCC ability (*Koren* et al. 1979) paralleled by reduction in NK susceptibility (*Gidlund* et al., to be published).

---

cytolysis using "cold", unlabeled tumor cells at various stages of differentiation did reveal that the reduction in lytic susceptibility linked to differentiation was in some systems indeed caused by a poorer binding ability and not via an increased resistance towards the lytic machinery of the NK cells. Analysis of cloned tumor lines undergoing such differentiation should not allow a more precise delineation of the specificity structures involved causing the decrease in NK susceptibility.

Specificity of mouse NK cells was shown to be dependent on actively produced trypsin-sensitive "receptors" on the outer surface of these cells (*Roder* and *Kiessling* 1978). The possibility remains, however, that at least part of "NK activity" may occur as a secondary feature endowed on the NK cells by IgG antibodies produced by B cells as suggested by results from the human system. Thus, NK cells have been shown to function well in ADCC systems (*Ojo* and *Wigzell* 1978) in parallel to their "own" specific lytic system. Whereas it would thus seem clear that NK cells can function on their own to provide their typical specificity profile(s), it can also be concluded that in certain situations significant lytic activity of a presumedly NK nature may in fact be manufactured by NK cells, but the specificity involved may be of antibody nature. This may in certain systems yield significant confusion to the analysis, since several target cells with only "low" NK susceptibility can be shown now by IgG coating to behave like highly NK susceptible targets (*Ojo* and *Wigzell* 1978). Judging from the evidence published so far, specificity problem of this nature due to precoating of NK cells with IgG may be more important when the worker is dealing with human NK cells in comparison to murine NK cells, due to the higher avidity at the cellular level of the Fc receptors for IgG on the human NK cell. Attachment of the NK cell to the target cell may thus occur via several means, and it may well be that successful attachment (allowing a minimal critical time of binding) will be enough for NK cells to lyse virtually any target cell. Several features are thus known to contribute to the binding forces of NK cells for sensitive targets in a relatively nonspecific manner. Charge and hydrophobicity of the potential target cell have thus been shown to be of significant importance in producing susceptible targets (*Becker* et al. 1979).

Also, work carried out with an NK-resistant variant of the NK-sensitive lymphoma L1210 have pointed to an intriguing correlation between high NK sensitivity and expression of the neutral glycolipid asialo-GM 2 (*Durdik* et al. 1980). In agreement with this result, we have recently observed a similar correlation between high NK sensitivity and expression of asialo-GM 2 when working with various variants and hybrids of the YAC-1 lymphoma. (Fig. 1a; from a collaborative study with *Yogeeswaran* and *Welsh*). In the same study we found indications that the amount of sialic acid released by neuraminidase seemed to correlate inversely with NK sensitivity among a panel of YAC-1 variants and hybrids (Fig. 1b), suggesting a protective role of sialic acid in the NK system. Clearly, these studies underline the possible influence of several molecules on NK sensitivity, which may not directly be involved as specific target structures. It is interesting to note, however, that long before the discovery of NK cells several authors suggested that sialic acid on the tumor cell surface may act as a barrier to the detection of antigens by the host organism (*Currie* and *Bagshawe* 1968).

There are, however, reports of macromolecules of a more defined nature displaying selective inhibitory capacity for NK cells in target binding assays (*Roder* et al. 1979b). This system showed a relatively complex pattern with species-specific as well as species-unrestricted molecules being involved (*Roder* et al. 1979). Availability of cloned NK cells and the use of soluble molecules for assessment of direct binding or inhibition of lysis would be required to ascertain these findings.

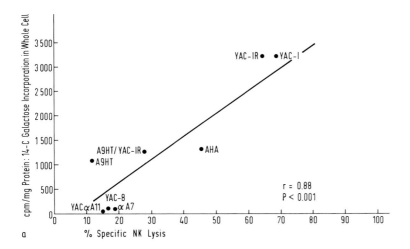

Fig. 1a. Correlation Between NK Sensitivity and Expression of Asialo-GM 2 Among YAC-1 Tumor Variants and Hybrids

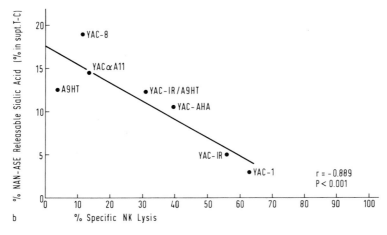

Fig. 1b. Correlation Between NK Sensitivity and the Amount of Neuraminidase Releasable Cell Surface Sialic Acid Among YAC-1 Tumor Variants and Hybrids

It is, however, clear that NK cells display in part a species-restricted (or species-preferred) lytic pattern (*Hansson* et al. 1978). This statement requires the use of several criss-cross studies using at the same time NK cells from two or more species and testing simultaneously against targets from the respective species. Using such assays we have repeatedly found that human NK cells are better lytic effector cells against human targets than mouse targets and vice versa for murine NK effector cells (*Hansson* et al. 1978; *Axberg* et al., to be published). However, within the various tumor/target systems analyzed one may find several individual tumors failing to disclose such species-preferential behavior. Furthermore, the use of proteolytic enzymes to pretreat the respective target cells before NK lysis has frequently yielded results indicating that species-restricting elements are preferentially eliminated from the target surface upon such treatment (*Axberg* et al. 1979). For example, as shown in Table 4 in a summary form, when two such tumors (murine

Table 4. Species preference of NK cells can be eliminated at the target level using trypsin treatment

| Effector cells[a] | Target cells[b] | | | |
|---|---|---|---|---|
| | YAC, normal | YAC, trypsin-treated | Molt 4, normal | Molt 4, trypsin-treated |
| Murine NK cells | ++++ | ++ | ++ | ++ |
| Human NK cells | ++ | ++ | ++++ | ++ |

[a] Normal murine spleen cells or normal human PBL:s. Independent surface markers and other criteria have established the NK nature of the effector cells. Assay short-term (4 h) 51-Cr release assay

[b] YAC is a murine Moloney T lymphoma. Molt–4 is a human T lymphoma. Trypsin treatment before the in vitro lytic assay using 0.25% trypsin for 45 min. +, susceptibility in relative terms. Reduction from ++++ to ++ means at least a two fold reduction in sensitivity. Details of assay can be obtained from *Axberg* et al. (1980)

and human T lymphomas, YAC-1 and Molt-4, respectively) were treated with trypsin before NK lysis only the lytic activity of NK cells derived from the same species was reduced in their lytic activity. It is clear that further genetic and biochemical analysis of target cells (or hybrid targets between human and murine NK-susceptible targets) are required to pinpoint the actual molecular basis of these specificity profiles. It is of course tempting to speculate that NK cells may represent a primordial primitive form of self-defense compared to the T/B lymphocyte systems and may well use a primitive MHC-like system to yield this species preference. Since NK cells in several other surface features behave as if they belong to the same or similar lineage as T lymphocytes, one may venture a guess that this species preference of NK cells could have the same underlying basis which is yielding a species preference with regard to the binding of T cells to certain cells in vitro (*Galili* et al. 1978).

Arguments on NK cell specificity in relation to clonally distributed receptors with specificity for diverse target structures will only be settled in a conclusive manner upon the availability of cloned cells in vitro with "accepted" NK cell nature. Reports on such cell lines behaving like NK cells do already exist, but so far have yielded unconclusive results as to whether these lines will display the usual NK profile when tested against a panel of target cells (*Dennert* 1980) or whether they rather will display a specificity of a much more restricted nature (*Nabel* and *Cantor*, personal communication). *If* clones of NK cells can be established which display the identical lytic activity against accepted NK targets within and across the species barrier as would normal spleen NK cells, this would constitute a powerful argument against the clonal theory of NK specificity. Yet, even such a finding would not exclude the possibility that some NK cells may differentiate into more specific cells with regard to specificity and may well then take into use similar genetic systems, i.e., T cells, when generating such new specificity patterns. If this can be shown to be true, one may well consider such activated, specialized "NK cells" to constitute a missing link in the phylogeny of the sophisticated killer T cells.

# 4 Concluding Remarks

In the present article we have refrained from making a complete coverage of NK cells as to features and functions. Two topics have been selected by us to be covered in more detail, namely, the in vivo relevance of NK cells and the problems about NK specificity. It should be clear for the reader that both issues are relevant yet in large areas unsolved. However, we deem it quite clear that since the discovery of NK cells as a distinct cell type the in vivo findings have by and large supported the hope that these cells may play a significant role in resistance toward malignant cells. Under exactly what situations NK cells may function to reduce or eliminate malignant cells originating in vivo is still, however, a matter to be further explored. The distribution of NK activity within the various lymphoid organs shows a striking and unique pattern of distribution, being high in blood and spleen but low in bone marrow and thymus (*Kiessling* et al. 1975b). We have previously ventured the concept that this distribution profile may either describe the actual distribution of NK cells as such in the various populations or, alternatively, be caused by normal cells with affinity for NK cells causing something like a "cold target" inhibition in the organs with low NK activity (*Kiessling* and *Wigzell* 1979). Support for such an idea has been accumulating over the last few years as several normal, particularly "embryonic" or primitive cell types can be shown to display significant susceptibility to NK lysis in vitro. Such normal NK-susceptible targets have indeed predominantly been found in the thymus and the bone marrow as discussed in this article. Thus, the fact that NK cells originally were found via their lytic ability toward malignant cells of certain types in vitro may have overshadowed the other role of these cells in relation to nonmalignant cells. The NK cells may thus serve as a possible regulator of distribution of hemopoiesis within the body in a similar way as they may reject retransplantation of bone marrow cells under certain circumstances (*Kiessling* et al. 1977). One may speculate that overactive NK cells under certain circumstances may down-regulate normal bone marrow functions in quite a significant manner. The fact that NK cells are actively regulated by interferons (*Trinchieri* et al. 1977; *Gidlund* et al. 1978) and the suggestions that NK cells are involved in providing resistance toward certain infections also add up to the conclusion that NK cells may be involved at several levels of immune defense.

*Acknowledgements*. Swedish Cancer Society, NIH Grant CA 26782-01 and NIH Grant CA 26752-01.

# References

Andersson LC, Jokinen M, Gahmberg CG (1979) Induction of erythroid differentiation in the human leukemia cell K562. Nature 278:364–365

Axberg I, Gidlund M, Örn A, Wigzell H (1980) Natural killer cells: notes on features and functions. In: Aiuti F, Wigzell H (eds) Serono symposium, thymus, thymic hormones and T lymphocytes 38:155–164

Axberg I, Zöller M, Wigzell H (to be published) Species restriction of NK cells studied at the level of the target cells

Becker S, Fenyo EM, Klein E (1976) The "natural killer" cell in the mouse does not require H-2 homology and is not directed against type or group-specific antigens of murine C-viral proteins. Eur J Immunol 6:882–888

Becker S, Stendahl O, Magnusson K (1979) Physico-chemical characteristics of tumor cells susceptible to lysis by natural killer (NK) cells. Immunol Commun 8:73–80

Brodt P, Gordon J (1978) Anti-tumor immunity in B lymphocyte-deprived mice. I. Immunity to a chemically induced tumor. J Immunol 121:359–367

Brodt P, Gordon J (to be published) Anti-tumor immunity in B lymphocyte-deprived mice. II. In vitro studies. J Immunol

Chernyakhovskaya IY, Slavina EG, Svet-Moldavsky GJ (1970) Antitumor effect of lymphoid cells activated by interferon. Nature 288:71–74

Chow DA, Greene MI, Greenberg AH (1979) Macrophage-dependent NK-cell-independent "natural" surveillance of tumors in syngeneic mice. Int J Cancer 23:788–797

Cudkowicz G (1968) Hybrid resistance to parental grafts of hematopoietic and human lymphoma cells. In: The proliferation and spread of neoplastic cells. Williams & Wilkins, Baltimore, p 661

Currie GA, Bagshawe KD (1968) The role of sialic acid in the antigenic expression: further studies of the Landschutz ascites tumour. Br J Cancer 22:843–853

Dennert G (1980) Cloned lines of natural killer cells. Nature 287:47–49

Dennert G (to be published) Cultivation of mouse NK cell lines in vitro. Nature

Dent PB, Fish LA, White JF, Good RA (1966) Chediak-Higashi syndrome. Observations on the nature of the associated malignancy. Lab Invest 15:1634–1642

Durdik J, Beck B, Clark E, Henney C (1980) Characterization of a lymphoma cell variant selectively resistant to natural killer cells. J Immunol 125:683–688

Galili U, Galili N, Vanky F, Klein E (1978) Natural species restricted attachment of human and murine T lymphocytes to various cells. Proc Nat Acad Sci USA 75:2396–2442

Gallin JI, Bujak JS, Patten E, Wolff SM (1974) Granulocyte function in the Chediak-Higashi syndrome of mice. Blood 43:201–206

Gidlund M, Örn A, Pattengale P, Wigzell H, Nilsson K (to be published) Induction of differentiation in two human tumor cell lines is paralleled by a decrease in NK susceptibility

Gidlund M, Örn A, Wigzell H, Senik A, Gresser I (1978) I. Enhanced NK cell activity in mice injected with interferon and interferon inducers. Nature 273:759–775

Gorelik E, Fogel M, Feldman M, Segal S (1979) Differences in resistance of metastatic tumor cells and cells from the local tumor growth to natural killer cells. J Nat Cancer Inst 63:1397–1403

Haller O, Wigzell H (1977) Suppression of natural killer cell activity with radioactive strontium: effector cells are marrow-dependent. J Immunol 118:1503–1506

Haller O, Hansson M, Kiessling R, Wigzell H (1977) Non-conventional natural killer cells may play a decisive role in providing resistance against syngeneic tumor cells in vivo. Nature 270:609–611

Hanna N, Fiddler I (to be published) The role of natural cytotoxic cells in the destruction of circulating tumor emboli. J Nat Cancer Inst

Hansson M, Kärre K, Bakacs T, Kiessling R, Klein G (1978) Intra- and interspecies reactivity of human and mouse natural killer (NK) cells. J Immunol 121:6–12

Hansson M, Kärre K, Kiessling R, Roder JC, Andersson B, Häyry P (1979a) Natural NK cell targets in the mouse thymus: characteristics of the sensitive cell population. J Immunol 123:765–773

Hansson M, Kiessling R, Andersson B, Kärre K, Roder J (1979b) Natural killer (NK) cell sensitive T-cell subpopulation in the thymus: inverse correlation to NK activity of the host. Nature 278:174–176

Hansson M, Kiessling R, Andersson B (1981) Human fetal thymus and bone marrow contain target cells for natural killer cells. Europ J Immunol 11:8–12

Harmon RC, Clark E, O'Toole C, Wicker L (1977) Resistance of H-2 heterozygous mice to parental tumors. I. Hybrid resistance and natural cytotoxicity to EL-4 are controlled by the H-2D-Hh-1 region. Immunogenetics 4:601–610

Herberman RB, Nunn ME, Holden HT, Lavrin DH (1975a) Natural cytotoxic reactivity of mouse lymphoid cells against syngeneic and allogeneic tumors. II. Characterization of effector cells. Int J Cancer 16:230–237

Herberman RB, Nunn ME, Lavrin DH (1975b) Natural cytotoxic reactivity of mouse lymphoid cells against syngeneic and allogeneic tumors. I. Distribution of reactivity and specificity. Int J Cancer 16:216–229

Herberman RB, Nunn ME, Holden HT (1978) Low density of Thy-1 antigen on mouse effector cells mediating natural cytotoxicity against tumor cells. J Immunol 121:304–309

Herberman RB, Deje JY, Kay HD, Ortaldo JR, Riccardi C, Bonnard GD, Holden HT, Fagnani R, Santoni A, Puccetti P (1979) Natural killer cells: characteristics and regulation of activity. Immunol Rev 44:43–70

Jensen P, Koren H (1979) Depletion of NK by cellular immunoadsorbtion. J Immunol 123:1127–1132

Kärre K, Klein GO, Kiessling R, Klein G, Roder JC (1980) Low natural in vivo resistance to syngeneic leukemias in natural killer deficient mice. Nature 284:624–626

Kasai JC, Leclerc JC, McVay-Bodreau L, Shen FW, Cantor H (1979) Direct evidence that natural killer cells in nonimmune spleen cell populations prevent tumor growth in vivo. J Exp Med 149:1260–1264

Kiessling R, Wigzell H (1979) An analysis of the murine NK cell as to structure, function and biological relevance. Immunol Rev 44:165–208

Kiessling R, Klein E, Wigzell H (1975a) Natural killer cells in the mouse. I. Cytotoxic cells with specificity for mouse Moloney leukemia cells. Specificity and distribution according to genotype. Eur J Immunol 5:112–117

Kiessling K, Klein E, Pross H, Wigzell H (1975b) Natural killer cells in the mouse. II. Cytotoxic cells with specificity for mouse Moloney leukemia cells. Characteristics of the killer cell. Eur J Immunol 5:117–121

Kiessling R, Petranyi G, Klein G, Wigzell H (1975c) Genetic variation of in vitro cytolytic activity and in vivo rejection potential of non-immunized semi-syngeneic mice against a mouse lymphoma line. Int J Cancer 15:933–940

Kiessling R, Petranyi G, Klein G, Wigzell H (1976) Non-T-cell resistance against a mouse Moloney lymphoma. Int J Cancer 17:1–7

Kiessling R, Hochman PS, Haller O, Shearer GM, Wigzell H, Cudkowicz G (1977) Evidence for a similar or common mechanism for natural killer cell activity and resistance to hemopoietic grafts. Eur J Immunol 7:655–663

Kirchner H, Hirt HM, Becker H, Munk K (1977) Production of an antiviral factor by murine spleen cells after treatment with *Corynebacterium parvum*. Cell Immunol 31:172–179

Klein G, Klein G, Kiessling R, Kärre K (1978) H-2 associated control of natural cytotoxicity and hybrid resistance against RBL-5. Immunogenetics 6:561–569

Koren HS, Andersson SJ, Larrick JW (1979) In vitro activation of a human macrophage-like cell line. Nature 279:328–330

Lam KM, Linna L (1979) Transfer of natural resistance to Mareks disease (JMV) with non-immune spleen cells. Studies of cell population transferring resistance. Int J Cancer 24:662–667

Loutit JF, Townsend KM, Knowles JF (1980) Tumor surveillance in beige mice. Nature 285:66–69

Möller G (ed) (1979) Natural killer cells. Immunol Rev 44

Nunn ME, Herberman RB, Holden HT (1977) Natural cell-mediated cytotoxicity in mice against nonlymphoid tumor cells and some normal cells. Int J Cancer 20:381

Ohno A, Amos DB, Koren HS (1977) Selective cellular natural killing against human leukemic T cells and thymus. Nature 266:546–548

Ojo E, Wigzell H (1978) Natural killer cells may be the only cells in normal mouse lymphoid cell populations endowed with cytophilic ability for antibody-coated tumor target cells. Scand J Immunol 7:297–305

Petranyi G, Kiessling R, Povey S, Klein G, Herzenberg L, Wigzell H (1976) the genetic control of natural killer cell activity and its association with in vivo resistance against a Moloney lymphoma isograft. Immunogenetics 3:15–28

Pross H, Gupts S, Good RA, Baines MG (1979) Spontaneous human lymphocyte-mediated cytotoxicity against tumor targets. VII. The effect of immunodeficiency disease. Cell Immunol 43:160–175

Reid LM, Jones C, Minato N, Bloom BR, Holland J (1979) Rejection of virus persistently infected tumor cells. I. Rejection in athymic mice. J Exp Med 149:1117–1123

Riccardi C, Santoni A, Barlozzari T, Puccetti P, Herberman RB (1980) In vivo natural reactivity of mice against tumor cells. Int J Cancer 25:475–486

Riccardi C, Barlozzari T, Santoni A, Herberman RB, Cesarini C (1981) Transfer to cyclophosphamide treated mice of natural killer (NK) cells and in vivo natural reactivity against tumors. J Immunol 126:1284–1289

Riesenfeld I, Örn A, Gidlund M, Axberg I, Alin G, Wigzell H (1980) Positive correlation between in vitro and NK activity and in vivo resistance towards AKR lymphoma cells. Int J Cancer 25:399–403

Roder JC, Kiessling R (1978) Target-effector interaction in the natural killer cell system. I. Covariance and genetic control of cytolytic and target-cell-binding sub-populations in the mouse. Scand J Immunol 8:135–144

Roder JC, Duwe AK (1979) The beige mutation in the mouse selectively impairs NK cell function. Nature 278:451–453

Roder JC, Kiessling R, Biberfeld P, Anderson B (1978) Target effector interaction in the natural killer cell system. II. The isolation of NK cells and studies on the mechanism of killing. J Immunol 121:2509–2517

Roder JC, Ährlund-Richter L, Jondal M (1979) Target-effector interaction in the human and murine natural killer cell system. Specificity and xenogeneic reactivity of the solubilized target structure complex and its loss in a somatic cell hybrid. J Exp Med 150:471–480

Roder JC, Lohmann-Matthes ML, Domzig W, Wigzell H (1979a) The beige mutation in the mouse. II. Selectivity of the natural killer (NK) cell defect. J Immunol 123:2174–2181

Roder JC, Rosén A, Fenyo EM, Troy FA (1979b) Target-effector interaction in the natural killer cell system: the isolation of target structures. Proc Natl Acad Sci USA 76:1405–1420

Roder JC, Haliotis T, Klein M, Korec S, Jett J, Ortlado J, Heberman RB, Katz P, Fanci AS (1980) A new immunodeficiency disorder in humans involving NK cells. Nature 284:553–556

Saksela E, Timonen T, Ranki A, Häyry P (1979) Morphological and functional characterization of isolated effector cells responsible for human natural killer activity to fetal fibroblasts and to cultured cell line targets. Immunol Rev 44:71–124

Seaman WE, Gindhart TD, Greenspan JS, Blackman MA, Talal N (1979) Natural killer cells, bone and the bone marrow: Studies in estrogen-treated mice and in congenitally osteopetrotic (mi/mi) mice. J Immunol 122:2541–2548

Sendo F, Aoki T, Boyse EA, Buofo CK (1975) Natural occurrence of lymphocytes showing cytotoxic activity to Balb/c radiation-induced leukemia RLo cells. J Nat Cancer Inst 55:603–610

Stern P, Gidlund M, Örn A, Wigzell H (1980) Natural killer cells mediate lysis of embryonal carcinoma cells lacking MHC. Nature 285:341–342

Stern P, Gidlund M, Kimura A, Wigzell H (to be published) Murine embryonal carcinoma cells functions as universal NK target cells

Talmadge JE, Meyers KM, Prieur DJ, Starkey JR (1980) Role of natural killer cells in tumor growth and metastasis in beige mice. Nature 284:622–623

Trinchieri G, Santoli D, Knowles B (1977) Tumor cell lines induce interferon in human lymphocytes. Nature 270:611–613

Troye M, Perlmann P, Pape GR, Spiegelberg HL, Näslund I, Gidlöf A (1977) The use of Fab fragments of anti-human immunoglobulin as analytic tools for establishing the involvement of immunoglobulin in the spontaneous cytotoxicity to cultured tumor cells by lymphocytes from patients with bladder carcinoma and from healthy donors. J Immunol 119:1061–1070

Warner NL, Woodruff MF, Burton RC (1977) Inhibition of the growth of lymphoid tumors in syngeneic athymic (nude) mice. Int J Cancer 20:146–155

Welsh R, Kiessling RW (1980) Natural killer cell response to lymphocytic choriomeningitis virus in beige mice. Scand J Immunol 11:363–367

Welsh RM, Zinkernagel RM (1977) Heterospecific cytotoxic cell activity induced during the first three days of acute lymphocytic choriomeningitis virus infection in mice. Nature 268:646–648

Windhorst DB, Padgett G (1973) The Chediak-Higashi syndrome and the homologous trait in animals. J Invest Dermatol 60:529–537

# Subject Index

# Of Further Interest from this Series

**Springer-Verlag**
**Berlin Heidelberg NewYork**

# Reviews of Physiology, Biochemistry and Pharmacology

Editors: R. H. Adrian, E. Helmreich, H. Holzer, R. Jung, O. Krayer, R. J. Linden, F. Lynen, P. A. Miescher, J. Piiper, H. Rasmussen, A. E. Renold, U. Trendelenburg, K. Ullrich, W. Vogt, A. Weber

## Volume 83

1978. 45 figures, 15 tables. IV, 196 pages
ISBN 3-540-08907-1

Contents: E. M. Wright: Transport Processes in the Formation of the Cerebrospinal Fluid. – L. B. Cohen, B. M. Salzberg: Optical Measurement of Membrane Potential. – L. Glaser: Cell-Cell Adhesion Studies with Embryonal and Cultured Cells. – P. Propping: Pharmacogenetics.

## Volume 84

1978. 23 figures, 2 tables. III, 240 pages
ISBN 3-540-08984-5

Contents: H. P. Godfrey, P. G. H. Gell: Cellular and Molecular Events in the Delayed-Onset Hypersensitivities. – E. Wintersberger: DNA Replication in Eukaryotes. – H. Z. Movat: The Kinin System: Its Relation to Blood Coagulation, Fibrinolysis and the Formed Elements of the Blood.

## Volume 85

1979. 64 figures, 7 tables. III, 231 pages
(58 pages in German).
ISBN 3-540-09225-0

Contents: M. Lindauer: Orientierung der Tiere in Raum und Zeit. –U. E. Nydegger: Biologic Properties and Detection of Immune Complexes in Animal and Human Pathology. – S. Matern, W. Gerok: Pathophysiology of the Enterohepatic Circulation of Bile Acids.

## Springer-Verlag
## Berlin Heidelberg New York

## Volume 86

1979. 44 figures, 3 tables. III, 206 pages
ISBN 3-540-09488-1

Contents:
P. Thorén: Role of Cardiac Vagal C-Fibers in Cardiovascular Control. – R. J. Hogg, J. P. Kokko: Renal Countercurrent Multiplication System. – P. Scheid: Mechanisms of Gas Exchange in Bird Lungs.

## Volume 87

1980. 26 figures, 6 tables. V, 232 pages
(8 pages in German)
ISBN 3-540-09944-1

Contents:
G. Moruzzi: In Memoriam Lord Adrian. – D. E. W. Trincker: Wilhelm Steinhausen. – U. Trendelenburg: A Kinetic Analysis of the Extraneuronal Uptake and Metabolism of Catecholamines. – J. T. Fitzsimons: Angiotensin Stimulation of the Central Nervous System. – L. D. Strawser, O. Touster: The Cellular Processing of Lysosomal Enzymes and Related Proteins.

## Volume 88

1981. 29 figures. V, 264 pages
(23 pages in German)
ISBN 3-540-10408-9

Contents:
R. Jung: Walter R. Hess 1881-1973. – K. M. Spyer: Neural Organisation and Control of the Baroreceptor Reflex. – M. Haider, E. Groll-Knapp, J. A. Ganglberger: Event-Related Slow (DC) Potentials in the Human Brain. – K. Starke: α-Adrenoceptor Subclassification.

## Volume 89

1981. 39 figures, 19 tables. V, 254 pages
ISBN 3-540-10495-X

Contents:
E. H. Heinz: Walter Wildbrandt. – P. D. Snashall, J. M. B. Hughes: Lunge Water Balance. – D. D. Bikle, R. L. Morrissey, D. T. Zolock, H. Rasmussen: The Intestinal Response to Vitamin D. – P. E. di Prampero: Energetics of Muscular Exercise.